STUDIES IN BIOETHICS

MORAL DILEMMAS
IN MODERN MEDICINE

STUDIES IN BIOETHICS

General Editor *Peter Singer*

Studies in Bioethics is a series aimed at introducing more rigorous argument into the discussion of ethical issues in medicine and the biological sciences.

MORAL DILEMMAS IN MODERN MEDICINE

Edited by
MICHAEL LOCKWOOD

Oxford   New York
OXFORD UNIVERSITY PRESS
1985

Oxford University Press, Walton Street, Oxford OX2 6DP

Oxford New York Toronto
Delhi Bombay Calcutta Madras Karachi
Kuala Lumpur Singapore Hong Kong Tokyo
Nairobi Dar es Salaam Cape Town
Melbourne Auckland

and associated companies in
Beirut Berlin Ibadan Nicosia

Oxford is a trade mark of Oxford University Press

First published 1985 as an Oxford University Press paperback
and simultaneously in a hardback edition

British Library Cataloguing in Publication Data
Moral dilemmas in modern medicine.—(Studies
in bioethics)
1. Medical ethics
I. Lockwood, Michael   II. Series
174'.2   R724
ISBN 0–19–217743–5
ISBN 0–19–286056–9 Pbk

Set by Hope Services
Printed in Great Britain by
Richard Clay (The Chaucer Press)
Bungay, Suffolk

For Gill

CONTENTS

INTRODUCTION

In March 1983 five Staff Tutors at the Oxford University
Department for External Studies, of whom I was one,* decided to
set up the Radcliffe Circle as a focus for our shared interest in the
social and ethical implications of science, medicine, and technology. We chose the name 'Radcliffe' since John Radcliffe
himself was a physician, and because, with the presence in
Oxford of a Radcliffe Infirmary, a John Radcliffe Hospital, and a
Radcliffe Science Library, the name seemed to have the right sort
of associations. Also, John Radcliffe's own empiricist and
pragmatic approach to medical science commended him to us.
The articles in this volume are essentially the edited texts of talks
given by invited speakers at a series of University seminars and
associated evening lectures which were arranged for Michaelmas
Term 1983 as a way of launching the Circle.

Both seminars and evening lectures were very well attended.
We were especially gratified by the very wide range of people that
came to them: at the seminars there were to be found students
and dons from practically every discipline. Clearly, we had struck
a chord. The seminars themselves were interdisciplinary in
character. Although five of the speakers are professional philosophers, lectures were also given by a lawyer and by three
practising doctors.

The large number of philosophers represented here no doubt
partly reflects a bias on my part, as organizer of the seminars, in
favour of my own discipline. Nevertheless, the philosophical
contributions to this volume may serve to alert people to the fact
that philosophers are now much more willing than in the recent
past to descend from their ivory tower and talk about 'real' issues.
The days when moral philosophers devoted most of their energies
to analysing the meaning of words such as 'right', 'good', 'duty',

* The other tutors involved in this initiative were Robert Elmore, John Durant,
Michael Shallis, and Geoffrey Thomas.

and so forth have gone. Philosophers are now perfectly prepared to tackle substantive moral questions, albeit in a way that is sensitive to subtle conceptual distinctions. But even today, few philosophers would think that time spent clarifying the meaning of the words they were employing was time wasted. Ordinary moral thinking is beset by an extraordinary amount of muddle, confusion, and unrecognized inconsistency: simply to get clear what the issues are is often to go a substantial way towards the satisfactory resolution of a moral problem. Actually, one of the best examples of this is to be found in this book in an article by someone who is, by profession, a lawyer rather than a philosopher: I refer to Ian Kennedy's discussion of the question whether doctors should be allowed, without either consulting or informing the parents, to prescribe contraceptives to under-age girls. Here the conceptual analysis and following through of logical implications seems to do most of the work, making the ultimate conclusion (controversial though it is) seem, in the light of the considerations he advances, well-nigh inescapable. Professional philosophers, it will be evident, have no monopoly on the analytical method.

Why has interest in medical ethics grown so rapidly in the last few years, both in Britain and elsewhere? It seems to me that there have been two, largely distinct, factors at work here, corresponding to two main focuses of concern. These might be dubbed, respectively, 'hi-tech angst' and 'the populist protest'. By 'hi-tech angst', I mean anxieties that derive, in one way or another, from the rapid pace of technological progress in medicine. It is felt that this progress has, in a number of ways, raised ethical problems for which traditional moral assumptions leave us unprepared. Modern 'hi-tech' medicine is now capable of keeping patients alive in circumstances in which they would previously have died *and in which it would generally have been considered a blessing that they should die*. Not for nothing was pneumonia once referred to as 'the old man's friend'; but pneumonia is now usually curable. When it becomes possible to keep alive, though often at enormous cost, patients who are suffering from severe senile dementia, are subject to pain so intense that they have to be drugged to the point of near in-sensibility, are terribly maimed, or are in a probably irreversible coma, the doctor is finding that the traditional imperatives of prolonging life and of doing what he judges best for his patients have been brought into sharp conflict with each other.

I mentioned cost. This itself raises a host of questions about priorities. Not only must society decide how much of its limited resources should be allocated to medicine, but, given that many modern medical techniques are so expensive and cannot therefore be made available to all who stand to benefit from them, doctors are faced with the morally extremely problematic question of whom to treat.

Finally, the exotic character of what medicine is now (or will be in the near future) in principle capable of providing raises problems of its own, once again finding us unprepared. There is still disagreement about the justification of such things as cosmetic surgery and sex-change operations, but the sense of moral disorientation is even greater when it comes to new, or projected, reproductive techniques: 'womb leasing', frozen embryos (or frozen-embryo orphans), gene therapy, growing human embryos in the laboratory to provide cell lines to treat diabetes (or even, more exotically still, using them to grow replacement organs), or choosing the sex or characteristics of one's child by way of sperm donation, genetic manipulation, or even 'cloning'. There is in this summary, as in the minds of most members of the public, a mishmash of serious science and what is likely, for a while, to remain science fiction. But even if we restrict ourselves to what is technically possible today, the possibilities are bizarre and, for many people, alarming. The Warnock Inquiry was set up in 1982 as a direct response to public concern about these matters; and Mary Warnock has contributed to this volume an article devoted to the discussion of some of the issues her Committee faced. I myself have included a paper, not given in the original lecture series (which preceded the publication of the Warnock Report), in which I examine some of the philosophical issues raised by the Report.

I dubbed the second main area of concern 'the populist protest'. We live, so we are told, in the age of the common man (or woman), in an era that is suspicious of 'élitism'. And this has prompted in many quarters a dissatisfaction with the extent to which doctors have been allowed, or at least are felt to have been allowed, to become a law unto themselves. Many people are beginning to feel that doctors, albeit usually with the best of motives, are too ready to keep their patients in the dark, make decisions on their behalf, and indeed abrogate to themselves powers that do not properly belong to them. This 'populist protest'—'more power for the patients'—is, of course, a pervasive theme in the writings of Ivan Illich. It also came through very strongly in Ian Kennedy's very influential 1980 Reith Lectures, *Unmasking Medicine* (reprinted from the *Listener* as *The Unmasking of Medicine* (London: Granada, 1983)). Usually the doctor, if so perceived, is thought of as at least a benign despot; though of course benign despotism is despotism for all that. But there are anxieties about whether it is invariably benign: I have in mind the fear that doctors may sometimes subordinate the patient's interest in getting the most promising available treatment to that of some research project or clinical trial. (This concern, which is reflected in Professor Hare's contribution to this volume, was itself the subject of a very influential book, *Human Guinea Pigs*, by M. H. Pappworth (London: Routledge and Kegan Paul, 1967), the title of which is deliberately echoed in that of Hare's article.)

It is a common criticism of doctors that they are apt to behave in a 'paternalistic' manner towards their patients; there is much talk, nowadays, of the need for 'informed consent' and of the necessity of 'respecting the patient's autonomy'. Four of the papers in this volume, those by Dr Muir Gray, Dr Raanan Gillon, Professor Kennedy, and Dr Roger Higgs, are concerned, in one way or another, with paternalism and autonomy. Professor Hare's paper, too, has a connection with these issues: the main problem about experimenting on children is precisely the fact that, at least when very young, they cannot be treated as fully autonomous agents capable of giving informed consent. It is a striking fact that all three of the doctors who have contributed to this book think that the issues of paternalism and autonomy are of crucial importance in their professional lives. These notions raise, however, some of the most difficult and fundamental questions in moral philosophy—questions, moreover, on which philosophers themselves are deeply divided.

There are two different ways of reasoning about morals. One way is what has come to be known as 'consequentialist': in choosing between different possible courses of action, one considers the overall goodness or badness of the states of affairs or sequences of events to which these actions will or may lead; as, for example, when one argues 'I shouldn't do this because it is likely to cause pain' (without presumably, sufficiently compensating benefits). The other form of reasoning involves an appraisal of the intrinsic character of the courses of action under consideration and, in particular, the extent to which they accord with various principles or precepts; as, for example, when one argues 'I shouldn't do this because it's dishonest.' These two forms of reasoning are not necessarily opposed to each other: some philosophers, of whom Hare is one, believe that these principles and precepts, and also the character traits we count as virtues, are, to the extent that they ought to guide our decisions, them- selves ultimately susceptible of justification in consequentialist (or even utilitarian) terms. But this is a highly controversial claim. And, even among 'consequentialists'—those who think that all that ultimately matters is what *happens* as a result of what one does—there are divisions of opinion about how the goodness or badness of states of affairs and events should be gauged. Should it be in terms of net enjoyment or suffering (as was believed by the classical utilitarians, such as Jeremy Bentham, John Stuart Mill, and Henry Sidgwick) or in terms of net desire fulfilment or non-fulfilment* (which is approximately what Hare believes) or in terms of a multiplicity of criteria that could include both of these along with justice, freedom, the advancement of knowledge, or what have you?

Precisely what line one takes on these highly theoretical matters can make a lot of difference to one's attitude towards, for example, autonomy or truth-telling and deception. For a start, is the requirement that the doctor should respect the patient's autonomy to be understood in consequentialist terms or in terms of what Robert Nozick calls a 'side constraint' on the doctor's behaviour? Should a doctor see his obligation, other things being equal, as that of promoting his patients' autonomy or of respecting their autonomous decisions? This may seem a rather subtle distinction, but it has substantial practical implications.

---

* These are distinct from enjoyment and suffering. Someone might want very much to be told if he was, say, terminally ill, realizing however that he would be likely to be happier, to suffer less, not knowing the truth.

Consider, for example, a severely depressed patient who refuses electro-convulsive therapy (ECT). Assume, for the sake of argument, that the patient is competent to make such a decision. Understanding his obligation to respect a patient's autonomy in the first of the two ways just distinguished, the doctor could argue as follows: 'The best way I know of promoting the patient's long-term capacity to act as a fully autonomous agent is to give him ECT. Therefore I am justified, *in terms of autonomy*, in overriding his autonomous decision, here and now, to refuse such treatment.' This is to argue in consequentialist vein. If the obligation to respect autonomy is understood in the second, non-consequentialist way, a doctor would not, in general, be entitled to override a patient's autonomous decisions about treatment, even for the sake of furthering that same patient's long-term autonomy. This extremely thorny issue, which has deep philosophical roots, arises quite independently both in Professor Kennedy's paper and in Dr Gillon's.

Assuming that we think of autonomy, in consequentialist terms, as a value to be promoted, a different but equally controversial question arises. Should we think of autonomy as valuable for its own sake, or rather as having derivative or instrumental value, for example as contributing to individual happiness? John Stuart Mill, as a self-proclaimed utilitarian, would seem to have been logically committed to taking it in the second way; but there are, notoriously, passages in his essay *On Liberty* that are difficult to construe other than as ascribing intrinsic value to individual autonomy.

Again, the stand that a doctor takes on this question may make a difference to his attitude if, for example, his patient has made an autonomous decision to refuse some treatment, without which his future health is likely to be in serious jeopardy. If autonomy is construed as something having independent value, then it can be weighed in the moral balance against considerations of the patient's welfare; if, on the other hand, autonomy is valuable only to the extent that it promotes the patient's welfare or happiness, it need not be thought of as having any moral weight where it is clearly at odds with that patient's health and happiness. There might still, however, be reasons for thinking that the welfare of society at large would be better served if doctors did not make too much of a habit of overriding patient's wishes 'for their own good'.

Then finally, of course, there is the difficult philosophical question of what exactly is meant by 'autonomy', what the capacity to make autonomous decisions consists in. Both Professor Kennedy and Dr Gillon devote a great deal of attention to this question.

Considerations similar to those I have just been surveying arise in many other contexts; in particular, they arise in connection with the question of honesty between doctor and patient. Just how much of a difference it might make to a doctor's behaviour in this regard if he was or was not a consequentialist, either of a utilitarian or non-utilitarian variety, I leave as an exercise for the reader.

A common complaint against philosophers is that they are good at raising questions, but not so good at resolving them. This is doubtless true in a sociological sense. They tend not to come up with answers that everyone, or even all philosophers, will agree with. But from that it does not follow that they never succeed in resolving the issue in the sense of arriving at the right answer. The contributors to this volume have a shared conviction that there is, in the end, no substitute in morals for rational argument—though it must, of course, be argument that proceeds from the right premisses, argument that is informed by an appropriate sensitivity to the matters at issue. Much as some philosophers inveigh against 'intuitionism', there will always be a point, in morals as elsewhere, where argument runs out and we can only appeal to what seems to us self-evidently correct. In this sense, as Dame Mary Warnock reminds us, sentiment too will always have a place in moral reasoning. 'Matters of ultimate value', as is remarked in the Warnock Report (echoing Mill), 'are not susceptible of proof.' Rational argument can only ever get us from our starting-point to our conclusion: and if our starting point is mistaken, so may our conclusions be, however impeccable our logic.

Some great thinkers of the past have thought that morals should be like geometry: that it should be a matter of applying incorrigible moral axioms to the given facts and then proceeding in linear fashion to a particular conclusion. Classical utilitarianism and Kant's 'deontological' ethics both appear to have been inspired by some such Cartesian ideal. But, for most contemporary thinkers, morals is a two-way street. We argue from principles to particular conclusions, certainly. But we also argue back from particular judgements to conclusions about matters of principle. As moral theorists, we seek a deeper-principled rationale for the particular moral judgements that we find ourselves disposed to make; and having provisionally arrived at such a rationale, we then explore its logical implications. Sometimes the explanatory power, economy, and inherent appeal of the principles we arrive at are such that we are prepared to discard particular judgements that they fail to sanction. At other times we take the fact that a principle has implications, in specific cases, which seem to us clearly unacceptable as grounds for modifying or discarding it.

This notion of passing back and forth between particular judgements and presumed underlying rationale, adjusting each in the light of the other until a satisfying harmony is arrived at, is a fashionable one nowadays. It is what the Harvard philosopher John Rawls refers to as the method of 'reflective equilibrium'. Yet even this, it seems to me, cannot be the whole story. Mere internal coherence and intuitive appeal can no more be a fully adequate criterion of correctness in moral theory than it is in science. It is not necessarily any advance to have succeeded in massaging one's prejudices into a logically consistent system. The discovery of strains and inconsistencies within our moral outlook is an important part of its internal dynamic; it is one of the things that makes it possible for us to change our views and, with luck, move forward. But even where there is already harmony and consistency, we ought to be ever open to the possibility that we are wrong; we ought to ask whether our views are a product of moral sensitivity or moral blindness. Sometimes, in morals, what is needed is not sharpened powers of reason, but a heightened, or otherwise altered, perception. What we need, on occasion, is not better arguments, but a new perspective.

Oxford   Michael Lockwood
Michaelmas Term 1984

1 WHEN DOES A LIFE BEGIN?[1]

MICHAEL LOCKWOOD

There is a tendency to think of philosophy, or at any rate philosophy as it is practised in Britain and America, as a subject with little direct practical application. This is doubtless true of much of what philosophers do, nor is it necessarily any bad thing. Certainly, very few philosophers practise their profession for the sake of any envisaged application. Nor should they, in my opinion. There is something philistine in the view that every human endeavour has to be useful. Understanding, clarity of thought, and philosophical insight, like knowledge and artistic achievement, ought to be regarded as intrinsically valuable. No doubt they will generally issue in considerable satisfaction, at least to certain individuals. But their value does not reside merely in their being a means to such satisfaction.

That said, however, there are certain questions which clearly have a large philosophical component, but on the answers to which matters of great practical moment turn. One such is the question when you or I first came into existence. Hardly a week goes by, these days, without some controversial issue in medical ethics erupting into the media. The central question frequently seems to be precisely that of when a human life begins, when a human being may be said to have come into existence. The abortion issue clearly hinges, in part, on this, as do the questions whether the 'morning after' pill is ethically acceptable, or whether it is morally permissible to throw away, freeze, or squash between glass plates for the purpose of microscopic observation, a live human embryo. Whilst it is clearly a good thing that public attention be focused on these issues, one cannot help but be struck by how little is achieved in the ensuing controversy. Not only is the discussion invariably inconclusive, it does not even seem to achieve the more modest end of clarifying the issue. It is more in the nature of a periodic muddying of already murky waters.

This essay is an attempt to prove to you that careful philosophical analysis is capable of shedding considerable light on a question such as this. I shall argue that there is a right answer to the question of when a human life begins, and that philosophical reflection can make a substantial contribution to revealing what that right answer is. This, I shall argue, is an area where philosophy can be of considerable practical value, even if that is not the main reason for doing philosophy.

One source of confusion in this debate is the rather careless bandying about of three notions which ought to be kept distinct from each other. These are the concepts of (a) a *living human organism* (in the rest of this paper I shall omit 'living' but it should be understood), (b) a *human being*, and (c) a *person*. For the purposes of this paper, 'human organism' is to be understood in a biological sense: a human organism is simply a (complete) living organism of the species Homo sapiens. 'Person', on the other hand, is not a biological concept at all. A person is a being that is conscious, in the sense of having the capacity for conscious thought and experiences, but not only that: it must have the capacity for reflective consciousness and self-consciousness. It must have, or at any rate have the ability to acquire, a concept of itself, as a being with a past and a future. Mere sentience is not enough to qualify a being as a person. But a person, in this sense, need not be human. Perhaps some non-human higher primates—chimpanzees for example—are persons in this sense; perhaps dolphins are. Probably there are persons, though not of course human persons, on planets of distant stars. Perhaps we shall one day be able to create persons artificially out of non-organic material (though it is not clear how we should know when we had done so; it is not behaviour that makes something a person, but rather the possession of an 'inner life' of the appropriate degree of richness and depth[2]).

I shall explain in a moment just how I intend to use the term 'human being'. First, however, I want to consider two fallacious, and indeed rather crude, arguments designed to show, respectively, that you and I came into existence at the moment of conception, and, on the contrary, that we came into existence much later than that, probably subsequent to birth. I have no idea whether either of these arguments has ever been put forward in the literature, at least in such a bald form; but that doesn't matter for my purposes. The first argument runs: You and I are human organisms; a human organism comes into existence at the moment of conception; therefore, we came into existence at the moment of conception. The second argument runs: You and I are persons; but a foetus is not a person; indeed, it seems likely that several months have to elapse before the new-born baby acquires any capacity for reflective consciousness or self-consciousness; therefore, it seems likely that we did not come into existence until some time after birth.

Both arguments are unsound. The first is valid, but its premiss is false. You and I are not human organisms. Consider the human organism corresponding to some given human being. If that human being were the very same thing as that organism, he would not only come into existence at the same time as the organism; he would also cease to exist at the same time as the organism ceased to exist. But hardly any reflective person believes this to be the case, at any rate invariably. Those who believe in the existence of an immortal soul do not believe this, because they believe that we continue to exist, even when the corresponding human organisms die, decay, and turn to dust. But those who do not believe in an immortal soul mostly do not believe either that the time at which a human being ceases to exist is necessarily the same as the time at which the corresponding organism dies. (I am assuming that a living human organism ceases to exist when it dies, so that a corpse is merely the remains of such an organism.) This is because most people are prepared to accept the concept of brain death. That is to say, most people accept that certain sorts of brain damage would constitute the end of our (mortal) existence, even if they did not prevent the continuation of such lower brain functions as are necessary to maintain respiration, circulation, and so forth. Suitable destruction of higher brain centres, coupled with the maintenance of such lower functions, would in most people's eyes mean that the living human organism remained, even though we were no more. That view now enjoys the status of scientifically educated common sense. I shall nevertheless attempt shortly to give a philosophical justification for it.

The second argument fails for quite different reasons. Its premiss is true, but not in such a sense as to support the conclusion drawn. Or at least, it has not been shown that it is true in the required sense. Consider the following parody of the argument: I am a philosopher; but the individual bearing my name in 1954 was not a philosopher; therefore, I did not exist in 1954. The point is that 'philosopher' is what is known as a 'phase sortal':[3] one and the same individual can be a philosopher at one time yet not be a philosopher at another earlier or later time. There are, on the other hand, some things which an object is, if at all, for the entire period of its existence, things which it cannot become or cease to be: we may call these *temporally essential* attributes. The property of being a building is in this sense temporally essential. You can reduce a building to a pile of rubble; but then the building no longer exists. Likewise, the building did not itself exist when the bricks of which it was composed had not yet been assembled. To cease to be a building is, for a building, to cease to be. Is personhood a temporally essential attribute of you or me? Personhood, that is to say, as I stipulatively defined it above. If it were, the second of our two arguments would be valid. Could I cease to be a person without ceasing to be? It seems pretty clear to me that I could. I want you to engage in the following thought experiment.[4] Suppose that you knew that you were going to suffer from a terrible disease, which would slowly extinguish your mental capacity for reflective consciousness or self-consciousness—those attributes that mark us off from at any rate most lower animals. But imagine that this disease still left the organism capable of sentience: it would still be aware, still be capable of experiencing sounds, colours, pleasure and pain, and so forth. Only higher cognitive functions would have gone. Now suppose this being were to be subjected to the most excruciating pain imaginable for some extended period. If you knew that it was going to be you that suffered the disease, and that it would be the brain you now possess, albeit pathetically reduced in cognitive capacity, whose pain centres were going to be stimulated, what would your attitude be towards the pain? Would you consider that it was going to happen to you? Would you deem it rational to fear this pain in a self-interested way? Or would you think of it as something that was going to happen to someone or something that was not, after all, you? So that, at most, you would view the prospect of this pain as you would view the prospect of it happening to a dog, say, of whom you were fond. If you think, as I do, that it would be rational to fear this pain in a self-interested way, then you will be forced to conclude that being a person is not a temporally essential attribute but merely a phase sortal. I could cease to be a person and yet still exist; and if so, then by the same token, it makes perfectly good sense to say that I did exist before I became a person, just as I existed before I became an adult, and existed before I became a philosopher. Some may disagree with this view. Some of you may think that it is not rational to fear the pain, in the example just given, as something that would be happening to you. All well and good: my point at the moment is just that it would not be absurd for someone to take the opposite view. If being a person is indeed a temporally essential attribute, that needs to be argued for; it is not obviously so, if indeed it is so at all.

One further point: some philosophers might accept that 'person' is merely a phase sortal, and that we existed, you and I, before we achieved personhood. Yet they might still insist that it is only when one becomes a person that one comes to have a serious right to life. If this human organism had been painlessly killed at birth then *a fortiori I* would have been killed, on this view. But, assuming that this did not violate anyone else's rights (for example, the mother's), that wouldn't have been a (seriously) wrong thing to do. That is a possible view. I shall have something to say about it later. At the moment, however, I am concerned not with the ethical issues, but rather with a substantive non-ethical philosophical question—albeit one that is widely thought to have important ethical implications.

The above discussion reveals that we need a term for whatever it is that you and I are essentially, what we can neither become nor cease to be, without ceasing to exist. I use the term *human being* to fill this slot. Some might think *conscious being* a better term: on the grounds that one could perhaps turn into a frog without ceasing to exist, but would then hardly be a *human* being, or on the grounds that the souls of the departed, if such there be, have ceased to be *human* beings without ceasing to be, or that Pinocchio existed, as a conscious being, before he became human. On this view, 'human being' means a conscious being with a human body: and since in principle one could acquire or cease to possess a human body without ceasing to be, '*human* being' is really just a phase sortal. Perhaps. But I shall ignore these niceties: there is a point beyond which pedantry ceases to be profitable.

We have thus refined our question: it is the question 'When does a human being come into existence?' And we have seen this to be a different question from that of when a human organism comes into existence or when personhood is attained. How are we to set about answering this question? Well there is one thing that seems to me now quite obvious, something that should be obvious to anyone with a philosophical training, though I have never heard any philosopher say it; and indeed, it only occurred to me relatively recently. It is this: The question of when a human being comes into existence is really the same question as that of what constitutes the identity of a human being over time: the so-called problem of personal identity. And this is something about which philosophers, at least since Locke, have had a very great deal to say. Perhaps I'm exaggerating a little in saying that they're the same question. What I mean is this: If one was able to answer the familiar philosophical question: 'What is it that makes someone at one time the very same human being as someone at another time?', then one would be able also to answer the question 'What has to happen for a human being to have come into existence in the first place?' (What has to happen at or after conception, that is.) To answer the first question, one would have to stipulate some relationship that has to hold between human beings considered at two given times if they are to be the same human being. But if one knew that, one would be able to answer the second question as follows: Any given human being, *a*, considered at a time *t*, may be said to have come into existence at the earliest time *t'* at which there is an individual *b* that stands to *a* in the appropriate relationship. Briefly, if I know what relationship is constitutive of my identity through time, then I know that I came into existence at the moment when there first existed something that stands in that relationship to me now.

Our problem thus reduces to that of determining what that

relationship might be. Unfortunately, virtually every proposal that philosophers have come up with seems open to fairly decisive objections. Locke, for example (who uses the term 'man' for what we are calling 'human organism' and is careful to distinguish this from 'person') suggested, notoriously, that a human being at a later time is identical with a human being at an earlier time if and only if the later human being can remember at least one of the experiences had by the human being at the earlier time.[5] This is clearly wrong, as it stands, for reasons pointed out by Reid.[6] It would mean that if I can now remember my first day at Oxford twenty years ago, but not my first day at school in 1949, whereas on my first day at Oxford in 1963 I could still remember my first day at school in 1949, then I am now identical with the person in this body who came up to Oxford in 1963, and that that person was likewise identical with the person in this body who first went to school in 1949, but that I now am not identical with that latter person. This is impossible; for it is part of the logic of identity that if a is identical with b and b is identical with c, then a is identical with c: identity is what logicians call a *transitive* relation. Admittedly, there are grounds, brought forward by Derek Parfit in a celebrated article,[7] for thinking that what is really important, what we ought to care about, is not identity, precisely, but a weaker non-transitive relationship that he calls 'survival'. That notion comes in handy when one considers the possibility, perhaps actualized in operations that involve the cutting of the corpus callosum (the tissue joining the two hemispheres of the brain), of one human being dividing into two. But it surely should not be invoked in the case just imagined: for surely, the little boy that first went to school in 1949 has survived. He did not die off as memories of his doings faded, say in the mid 1970s. No, Locke is just wrong. It has been suggested that Locke's original criterion be modified, so that a human being, a, at a later time, is to be considered identical with a human being, b, at an earlier time, if either a, at the later time, can remember at least one of b's experiences at the earlier time, or else there is a chain of intermediate times, such that at each time there is a human being who can remember at least one of the experiences of a human being at the preceding time, and at the two end points of the chain we have human beings who can remember at least one of the experiences of *b*, and who has at least one experience that can be remembered by *a*, respectively.[8] This is what is known in the trade as 'taking the ancestral' of the relation that Locke originally proposed: the new relationship stands to the old just as 'ancestor of' stands to 'parent of'. There remains a bit of a problem about periods when one is unconscious, and therefore has no experiences, but surely still exists; but perhaps this can be got round counter-factually—by appealing to what would have been the case had one been awake. But let us waive that problem. It does seem clear that, if this new proposal were correct, it would provide a basis for answering the question of when a human being comes into existence. I, presumably, would have come into existence at the earliest time at which there was associated with this body an experience which is joinable to my present experiences by a memory chain such as that just described. Subject to a certain vagueness about just what counts as remembering, this would seem to be a matter of scientific fact—no doubt difficult to determine, perhaps impossible to determine precisely, but a matter of fact nevertheless. At this point, the philosopher could bow out in favour of the child psychologist or perhaps the neurophysiologist, once the physical basis of memory is better understood.

I have put all of this in the subjunctive mood, since I do not in fact believe that this new proposal is correct. For one thing, it fails to cater for total amnesia. If the descent of a roof-tile on to my head or a series of electric shocks through the brain were to have the effect of 'wiping the tapes', erasing all memories of past experiences beyond recall, it seems to me I would still exist. Consider this. First I tell you that I am going to torture you to death. Then I tell you that I shall erase your memories first. Are you at all relieved? Do you think that it will not be you that is tortured to death? I don't. Indeed, there seems to me to be something fundamentally misconceived about the whole way in which Locke, and most of his successors, approach the problem of personal identity. In a way, I think they're mistaken about what sort of problem it is. Philosophers characteristically write about the issue as though it were a matter of finding the right *definition* of the phrase 'is identical with' as applied to human beings at different times. I don't think it is. I think it is a matter of fact, not definition, what the continuing identity of a human being through time consists in.

Consider the following two imaginary cases. Case 1. You are in hospital suffering from an inoperable brain tumour. The prognosis is exceedingly bleak; the doctors are clearly very worried. Then one day, the consultant comes to your bedside surprisingly cheerful. 'I think', he says, 'we might be able to do something for you, after all.' Hope surges within your breast. 'Yes', the consultant continues, 'we've made a lot of progress lately in microsurgical techniques enabling us to suture ruptured nerve fibres. Indeed, we can do this, in suitable cases, even with fibres coming from different individuals. We've been experimenting with animals; and we're now ready to try the technique on a human being. In another ward, we have a very sad case of a woman involved in a car accident. Her body is hopelessly smashed up; but we've been able to maintain a supply of blood to her brain. We now intend, with your consent, to give you a new brain—by transplanting her brain into your skull.' How do you react? Do you think: 'Gosh, I'm going to live after all'? No. The doctor is surely wrong. What he is proposing is not so much giving you a new brain as giving the accident victim a new body. Transplanting the woman's brain into your skull is fine for her (though if you're a man, it might create problems of adjustment), but it will do nothing for *you* at all. You are still going to die—even sooner, in fact, assuming that your brain is to be discarded after the operation.

Now consider another case, only more fantastic. Case 2. Freddy Laker, trying to make a come-back after the collapse of his Skytrain operation, announces a splendid new way of crossing the Atlantic. It's much simpler than anything yet devised. He has set up a series of booths on Victoria Station. What you do is step into a booth, insert your credit card, which is promptly returned to you, and dial your intended destination—say, New York, Chicago, Dallas, or San Francisco. Assume you choose New York. You press a button and . . . whoosh! You find yourself standing in a somewhat similar booth in Grand Central Station on Park Avenue. This, at any rate, is the claim. And several people who have already tried it attest that it really works. It is relatively cheap and involves none of the hassle that surrounds conventional air travel. It rapidly becomes *the* way to travel. You, who haven't yet travelled this way, are invited to attend a conference in San Francisco, and are tempted to use the new Laker service. But you are curious about just how it works. You make enquiries and learn that the principle is as follows. When the button is pressed, the body in the booth is scanned by an intense beam of high-energy radiation that maps the position and chemical constitution of every molecule in your body. This information is digitally recorded and beamed as a radio message, via satellite, to the corresponding booth in San Francisco, where a new body is almost instantaneously assembled, drawing on material from a molecule bank. Meanwhile, the intensity of the scanning beam has had the effect of vaporizing the original body. It is hardly surprising that the person finding himself in the booth in San Francisco should possess all the memories of the person who stepped into the booth on Victoria Station, and indeed, have the impression that he was, a moment ago, in London, given that the two bodies are, as near as makes no difference, qualitatively identical down to the last molecule. But is the person who steps out of the booth in San Francisco right in thinking that *he* was, a moment ago, in London? Is it really the same person? Is this, in fact, a neat way of crossing the Atlantic, or just a rather bizarre way of committing suicide?[9] Now you will doubtless be able to find some philosophers who at an impressionable age have been made to read Locke and his successors, who will insist that it is the same human being who both steps into the booth in London and subsequently steps out of the booth in San Francisco. But what do *you* think? What do you think intuitively? It seems to me quite clear that if I were to step into the booth in London, what would step out of the booth in San Francisco would not be me, but a newly created individual possessed of the illusion of being me. (Of course, if it was me that stepped into the original booth, then, given that I knew the facts about how the system worked, the individual stepping out of the other booth wouldn't actually *think* that he was me, since he would be bound to share my philosophical convictions.) If this seems unclear to you, imagine now that Freddy Laker were to develop a Mark 2 model, that could work the same trick with a less intense beam of radiation, that left the original body intact. Then almost everybody would come to see that even the original device was not, as it purported to be, a 'tele*transporter*', but merely a human being duplicator. Nobody, I take it, would think that the identity of what comes out the other end can depend on whether or not the original body remains. (To say, as some philosophers might, that this latter was a case of one human being *splitting* into two seems to me desperately implausible.) In short, I put it to you that what emerges at the other end is merely a copy, not the original article. If I am right about that, then it would show that continuity of memory, indeed psychological continuity generally, is not only not a necessary condition of continuing identity, as is shown by the amnesia example, but that it is not a sufficient condition of continuing identity either. For clearly the person who emerges from the booth in San Francisco does stand in Locke's relation to the person who enters the booth in London.

What both these examples seem to me to suggest is that a human being cannot be me unless he has my brain, or at any rate some crucial part of my brain. That is why *I* want to insist that the individual emerging from the booth in San Francisco is not me: he doesn't have *my* brain. Of course, he has a brain that is qualitatively indistinguishable from mine, but that isn't good enough. A fake Rembrandt is still a fake, even if it is a perfect copy of a genuine Rembrandt; a copy is still a copy, even if it is a perfect copy. No power on Earth would induce *me* to use Freddy Laker's machine.

Assuming that all this is correct, it has immediate implications for the kinds of medical ethical dilemma that I cited at the beginning of this paper. Take, for example the recent controversies surrounding the 'morning after' pill and Robert Edwards's supposed mistreatment of human embryos a few days old.[10] The worry, in each case, stems from the fear that what is being destroyed or damaged is an innocent human being. That, on the present view, cannot be true. For newly fertilized human ova and week-old human embryos *do not yet have brains*. If the brain is what is crucial here, then we must conclude that, before the brain comes into being, there is no human being there to worry about. Of course, there is a potential for a human being. But then that is equally true of a sperm and an ovum before conception. Suppose we have sperm and an ovum in a Petri dish. We're observing through a microscope and find one sperm that is clearly just about to fertilize the ovum. We then, just in the nick of time, drop a glass partition between them to prevent fertilization taking place. Is there anything intrinsically wrong with that? Surely not; no more than there is with ordinary contraception. Yet there is a potential, here, for the coming into existence of a specific human being, which is thereby being prevented from being realized. But if the brain is what is important, then if it is not wrong to thwart this potential at that point, then no more is it wrong to thwart this potential at any later point before brain development. That, at least, seems to be the logical conclusion to draw. And indeed, a view very much like that seems to have been gaining ground recently (though actually it has been current in the literature at least since the mid 1960s: see below, note 20). The suggestion is that we should apply to the developing embryo a criterion of *brain life* (my term), as a basis for saying when a human being comes into existence, that is the symmetrical counterpart of the criterion of brain death, used for determining when a human being goes out of existence, or at least when soul and body may be presumed to part company. (An eloquent recent statement of this point of view is to be found in a letter by an American physiologist, Libet, published in the journal *Science* in 1981;[11] the view is also endorsed by Peter Singer and Deane Wells, in their book on *in vitro* fertilization and related matters.[12]) This proposal I believe to be fundamentally correct.[13]

But we are getting ahead of ourselves, philosophically speaking. As I remarked earlier, philosophers have traditionally seen the problem of personal (or perhaps we should really say 'human') identity as one of coming up with an acceptable definition or conceptual analysis. Now it is generally agreed that reference to the brain simply does not belong in any analysis of what is *meant* when one speaks of a given later human being as being identical with a given earlier one. It does not belong to the *concept* of personal identity. Aristotle, after all, presumably had the same concept of personal identity as we do, and meant the same by whatever Greek words would express that notion as we mean by the corresponding English words. Yet he, as is well known, considered that the brain was merely an instrument for cooling the blood. And there is another consideration. Many people believe that the self, the human being (or, at least, the conscious being) survives the death of the body and *a fortiori* that of the brain. There is, surely, nothing in that that runs contrary to what we *mean* by the continuing identity of a human being. (To be sure, there are some philosophers who think that materialism is somehow true by definition, a conceptual truth; but they've never succeeded in making out a plausible case.) Also, we have no difficulty in understanding science fiction stories in which people switch bodies, including their brains. For this reason, even materialistically minded philosophers have, for the most part, resisted accounts of personal identity that make essential appeal to what is really just a matter of scientific theory.

What I want to suggest here is that the question 'What do we mean when we speak of the identity through time of a human being?' and the question 'What does that identity actually consist in?' are two distinct questions, and that an answer to the first, supposing it could be given, would still leave the second unresolved. Consider the analogy (inspired by Saul Kripke[14]) of gold. (I was rather proud of having thought of this analogy, until I discovered that John Mackie uses precisely the same analogy in his *Problems From Locke* to make essentially the same point.[15]) The question 'What do we mean by "gold"?' clearly is not the same question as the question 'What does gold actually consist in? What is it about what we call "gold" that makes it gold?' The way the concept of gold functions is roughly as follows. We find a certain kind of stuff lying around—a stuff distinguished by certain readily discernible attributes. These would include yellowish hue, metallic, heavy, resists most acids but not aqua regia, excellent conductor of electricity, and so on. But these attributes do not make gold gold. The concept allows for the possibility that some quite distinct substance might possess all of these attributes and yet not really be gold: a kind of super fool's gold. No, the assumption is, and has always been, that what makes gold gold, what being gold actually consists in, is the possession by a stuff of the appropriate underlying nature, whatever that might be. (This point has been urged by a number of philosophers in the last decade or so, most notably Hilary Putnam[16] and Saul Kripke.) This underlying nature, when properly understood, would be expected to explain why, under normal conditions, gold displays the discernible attributes that it does. But at the same time, it is possible that something might have the right underlying nature to be genuine gold, and yet for other reasons, not display the attributes by which we normally recognize gold as gold. Perhaps there could be a state of gold in which it appears, for example, as a blue liquid. The same goes for any substance term. (That is why it was not absurd for Thales, the earliest philosopher of whose thought we have any record, to suggest that everything might be water.) In the light of recent scientific developments, we now think we know what underlying nature constitutes a given stuff as gold: it is the possession of the right atomic structure. Specifically, something is gold, it is now believed, in virtue of being made up of atoms with the atomic number 79. That, we now think, is what being gold actually consists in. That is what gold is as a matter of fact, not definition. (The scientists just conceivably could have got it wrong.)

Exactly the same, I believe, goes for personal identity. There is a variety of discernible continuities within the biography of a given human being. Memory is one: the capacity to remember, at later times, experiences had and actions performed at earlier times. But there are others: knowledge of facts and of skills, continuity of attitudes, of behavioural dispositions, and of character traits. These can change, of course. But they usually change gradually, and they certainly do not, as a rule, change suddenly all together. Further, there is a causal continuity. Later actions flow from earlier intentions. Later attitudes are explainable in terms of earlier occurrences and so forth. Also, we have an introspective awareness of continuity within ourselves, of which memory, long and short term, is perhaps the principle ingredient. What philosophers have tried to do is *define* personal identity (or some kindred notion such as survival) in terms of these discernible continuities—mostly in terms of memory, though some writers, most notably Parfit,[17] have appreciated the importance of the other continuities as well. But this I believe to be a mistake. It is mistaken for exactly the same reason that it would be a mistake to try to *define* 'gold' in terms of yellowness, malleability, and so forth. For our ordinary concept of identity through time of a human being is not of something that is *constituted* by these discernible continuities, but as something that *underlies* these continuities and accounts for them—something of which these discernible continuities are merely a manifestation. Just what this underlying continuity might consist in is left open in our concept of personal identity; it is left open as far as the *meaning* of the relevant words goes. Thus, it is open to someone to hold, as do most Christians, that what underlies the discernible continuities of human personality is ultimately an immaterial soul—a soul that survives the death of the body. That is a logical possibility; though I must admit that I see not the slightest reason for believing it to be true. The view that I favour, and that I think is favoured by the available scientific evidence, is that what underlies the discernible continuities of memory and personality is a continuity of physical organization within some part or parts of a living human brain persisting through time.[18]

If this is right, then our earlier, tentative conclusion is sustained. Just as I shall live only as long as the relevant part of my brain remains essentially intact, so I came into existence only when the appropriate part or parts of my brain came into existence, or more precisely, reached the appropriate stage of development to sustain my identity as a human being, with the capacity for consciousness. When I came into existence is a matter of how far back the relevant neurophysiological continuity can be traced. Presumably, then, my life began somewhere between conception and birth. Certainly not *at* conception, and certainly not before my brain came into being. A more precise determination would require more scientific knowledge than I possess and probably more than anyone possesses at present.[19] And ultimately, of course, the attempt to fix a precise point would founder, even against a background of scientific omniscience, on the imprecision of the concepts I've been invoking. 'Human being' is not itself a completely precise concept, and *a fortiori* nor is that of a human life. But nor is it so vague that absolutely any view on the question of when, between conception and early infancy, a life begins is philosophically sustainable.

The view I have put forward is, of course, materialistic in its general tenor. But, even so, I see no reason why those who prefer to believe in an immaterial soul should be hostile to a notion of brain life, parallel to the now familiar notion of brain death. Their view allows, as mine does not, for the *possibility* that, even before the development of the brain, there is a human being already ensconced in the developing foetus. But, as far as I can see, there is no positive reason whatever for them to hold that this is *actually* the case. In particular, I can see *no connection* between the Catholic position on these matters and the rest of Catholic theology. There does not seem to be a distinctively Catholic position on brain death.[20] But any Christian who feels that body and soul at least go their separate ways at brain death ought in consistency to hold that they come together only at the point when whatever is destroyed at brain death first comes into being.

What, then, of the ethical implications of all this? Well, in the first place, nothing whatever in the way of a moral conclusion will follow from what I have been saying without the addition of some suitable moral premiss. One cannot derive an 'ought' from an 'is'. But most people would accept that, other things being equal, it is wrong deliberately to kill an innocent human being. (Personally, I am inclined to think that it is somewhat wrong, other things being equal, deliberately to kill any sentient being, the degree of wrongness being a function, in part, of how far up the scale of awareness it is; but I shall not attempt to argue this here.) In the absence of other considerations, two things would appear to follow. First, unless the interests of some other being are affected thereby, it is morally permissible to do whatever one likes with a human embryo or foetus before brain development. And that will include aborting it or experimenting with it in the laboratory. One caveat must be added, however. What I have just said holds only under the assumption that the embryo or foetus is not going to be allowed to develop to the point where, according to the above line of argument, a human being comes into existence. It is clearly possible to do harm to human beings who do not exist yet, by suitably mistreating embryos or foetuses from which such human beings are going to derive. Thus it would be very wrong to arrange for conception in the laboratory, do something to the resultant embryo that meant that any human being it developed into would be born blind, and then reimplant it with the intention that it should so develop. The insistence, in the guidelines recently laid down by the British Medical Assocation,[21] that human embryos selected for experiment or prolonged observation of a kind that is likely to damage them should not then be reimplanted, obviously makes good sense.

What about abortions that take place after the point when, according to the present theory, a human being comes into existence? Does it follow from our premises that these should be forbidden? No. What certainly follows is that such abortions should not be lightly undertaken. It would probably follow that, to take a familiar example, it would be morally wrong for a woman to have an abortion merely so that she did not have to postpone a skiing holiday which she had planned. But it would always be possible for someone to argue that, whilst such abortions were *prima facie* wrong—since deliberately to kill an innocent human being is always *prima facie* a wrong thing to do—it might not be wrong all things considered. For there might be all kinds of countervailing considerations: likely handicap, difficulty of seeing that it received reasonable care, and the burden that we should be placing on the mother by insisting that she brought the child to term. This last is a very important consideration and has been made much of by Judith Jarvis Thomson in a celebrated article on abortion.[22] It is, I think, a feature of our ordinary moral thinking—at what Hare would call the 'intuitive level'[23]—that there is a limit to the degree of self-sacrifice that can reasonably be demanded of someone in the name of duty. Perhaps it is just too much to ask of a woman that she be made to endure the trauma of birth and the burden of pregnancy against her will, especially if there are contributory circumstances, such as extreme youth or rape, that make the whole business even more of an ordeal. What would seem logical, from the present standpoint, is a change in our present abortion law, so as to allow abortion on demand before the neural structures underlying consciousness have developed (say, within the first ten weeks[24]), but imposing more stringent conditions thereafter—such, for example, as those who drafted the present legislation actually had in mind. (It is clear that their intentions have been flouted.)[25] But to arrive at a clear-cut, rationally defensible position on all these matters would call for a far more extended discussion than we have time for.

I would, however, like to look briefly at an alternative ethical starting-point, alluded to above. According to some philosophers, including Michael Tooley[26] and, at one time, Peter Singer[27] (though I think I may have gone some way towards arguing him out of it[28]), only persons have a right, or a 'serious right', to life. Singer argues this on the basis that only persons have a preference for going on living. Now I think it is true that one of the things that makes it so wrong deliberately to kill an innocent adult human being is indeed that she or he may reasonably be expected to have, not only a strong desire to go on living, but also a host of other desires for the fulfilment of which continued life is a *sine qua non*. So I am prepared to concede that it may not be *as* wrong to kill a human being who lacks such preferences as to kill one that has them. It is presumably for this reason (possibly amongst others) that most doctors would think it right to save a mother in preference to her unborn child, in circumstances where they could only save one. In 1983 the Irish Parliament passed an amendment to their Constitution outlawing abortion; the fact that the wording of this amendment appeared to confer on the unborn child a right to life equal to that of its mother provoked considerable opposition, even amongst those who did not approve of abortion as such. But that said, there are lots of things that it is wrong to do to human beings, not because of any preference or desire on their part, but simply because so to act would run *contrary to their interests* (Parents, for example, who failed to send their children to school might not be acting contrary to their children's wishes or preferences, but would almost certainly be acting against their best interests.) A human being who has the potential to become a person has a very strong interest in being allowed to continue to live, assuming that we are agreed that being a person is a rather wonderful thing, and assuming also that the person in question will be reasonably content. That is why killing a new-born kitten, say, cannot be equated with killing a new-born infant, even if there is, at the time, little to choose between them in terms of their respective levels of awareness and cognitive capacities. If we value those attributes that mark us off, as adults, from the members of other species, then we are bound to admit that the new-born infant has much more to lose by being prematurely killed off. But we can still admit that it is less wrong to kill a new-born infant that lacks a preference for continued life than it would be to kill an adult who had such a preference. And that will explain why so many of us feel that Leonard Arthur was acting quite properly, from a moral standpoint, whereas to kill a Down's syndrome child of sixteen, say, would be unconscionable (unless it was so severely retarded as to enjoy a level of awareness no higher than that of a dog, say).

Common sense holds that it is very wrong deliberately to kill any innocent human being beyond earliest infancy, also wrong, but somewhat less wrong, to kill a new-born infant (the Greek practice of exposing unwanted new-borns disgusts us far less than the Maya and Inca practice of sacrificing adolescent girls), and not wrong at all to prevent a given sperm that would otherwise have done so from fertilizing a given ovum. Yet a surprising number of philosophers, amongst others Peter Singer, Michael Tooley, Jonathan Glover, and R. M. Hare, have felt obliged to embrace the counter-intuitive conclusion that there is nothing intrinsically to distinguish, morally, early infanticide from the mere prevention of conception.[29] For, on the one hand, neither a sperm-and-ovum-about-to-fuse, nor a new-born infant, actually possesses any of those attributes, such as rationality or reflective self-consciousness, that mark off most human beings from those lower animals that it is thought by most people (though mistakenly, in my estimation) morally permissible to kill (provided it is done humanely). But on the other hand both the new-born infant and the sperm-and-ovum have the potential to develop such attributes. So either potential counts, and prevention of conception, early infanticide, and abortion are (ignoring side effects) equally wrong; or else only the actual possession of such attributes as rationality and reflective self-consciousness counts, and early infanticide, abortion, and the prevention of conception are (again barring side effects) equally permissible, morally speaking. When these are seen to be the only alternative philosophically stable positions, it is hardly surprising that so many philosophers should plump for the second, unattractive and implausible though it seems. Actually, only Tooley thinks that, barring side-effects, deliberate failure to conceive, abortion, and infanticide are all equally permissible *tout court*; for Singer, Glover, and Hare, they are only permissible where they result in no net loss of utility: happiness for Singer, worthwhile life for

Glover, overall preference satisfaction for Hare. Ignoring social effects, and effects on others generally, 'newborn babies, like foetuses, are', according to Glover, 'replaceable. It is wrong to kill a baby who has a good chance of having a worth-while life, but . . . it would not be wrong to kill him if the alternative to his existence was the existence of someone else with an equally good chance of a life at least as worth-while . . . Just as it may be right to defer conception if later you stand a better chance of having a normal child, so . . . it can be right to kill a defective baby and then have a normal one you would not otherwise have.'[30]

I hope, however, to have shown that these are not the only philosophically viable positions, and that something much closer to the common-sense view is, after all, defensible. It is relatively unproblematic that the actual possession of rationality, reflective self-consciousness, and so on should count for more than their mere potential possession—or rather that their having been acquired should (reversibly comatose patients may possess them only potentially). That aspect of the common-sense position makes good sense, as we have seen, in terms of the moral weight to be attached to a desire for continued life, or for things for which that is a prerequisite. But as for potentiality—well there is potentiality and potentiality. To say that both a sperm about to fertilize an ovum and a new-born child have the potential to become a person is to ignore a crucial distinction between the two cases. A new-born child has the potential actually to *be* a person; if it becomes a person, that person is identical with, is the same human being as, the new-born child. Consequently, assuming that a person is a good thing to be, the new-born child has an interest in this potential being brought to fruition. And what goes for a new-born child also, I have argued, goes for a late foetus. But the sperm and ovum, in contrast, do not have the potential ever to be a person, but only to become a person in the more oblique sense of turning into a human organism, comprising a brain capable of sustaining a human life. And that, I have suggested, goes for the early embryo as well. If it develops normally, it will, to be sure, one day be a mature human organism to which there corresponds a person. But persons, as I argued at the beginning of this paper, are not identical with human organisms. Nor, therefore, is the embryo identical with the person that, in the sense just indicated, it becomes. And nor, correspondingly, does it have any interest in this potential being realized. Indeed, embryos, I would suggest, are not the sorts of things that can have interests at all. Nor are, strictly speaking, even mature human organisms: it is the corresponding human beings that have interests.

Thus there is all the difference in the world between killing a week-old embryo and killing a neonate. Neither may be a person. But the second is a human being, with an interest in continued life. When all that exists is the embryo, on the other hand, there is nothing there to have interests. You and I once were new-born infants; we were never week-old embryos, any more than we were sperm or ova or (except metaphorically) twinkles in our parents' eyes.

Postscript (February 1985)

Beings with the potential to enjoy worthwhile life have, so it was argued in the article, an interest in their own continued existence. Questions of identity are therefore crucial to determining the moral status of the human embryo or foetus. For we need to know whether the *very same being* that could later be said to be enjoying that worthwhile life yet exists. If it doesn't, then there is nothing there to have such an interest in its continued existence (or, indeed, in anything else). Couple this consideration with the thesis that what sustains human identity is a continuity of organization within a continuously existing brain. Assume, further, that only beings with interests are legitimate objects of moral concern. The conclusion is then plain: the human embryo, before brain development, is not, considered in itself, a legitimate object of moral concern.

That is what I argued in the foregoing article, and the line of reasoning seems to me as intellectually compelling now as when I wrote it (in October 1983). But it leaves a number of moral loose ends. Clearly there can, on this view, be nothing intrinsically wrong with experimenting on early human embryos, provided they are destroyed before brain development. But is there, on this view, anything *necessarily* wrong with experimenting on live human embryos or foetuses after the point at which, according to me, human life begins? Suppose, for the sake of argument, we assume (i) that the embryo or foetus has not been deliberately reared to this point for the purposes of providing an experimental subject (but has been aborted, say), (ii) it is not viable—there is no possibility of its surviving to term, (iii) the experiments in question cause no suffering, and (iv) there are no deleterious moral consequences for others, either in the long or short term. The question whether experimenting on the embryo or foetus is then open to moral objection hinges, in my view, on whether such experiments would run counter to the interests of the human being embodied in the embryo or foetus. On the face of it, it is difficult to see how it could; it cannot, seemingly, if a human being's interests are to be defined solely in terms of the quality of his life and the satisfaction or otherwise of his desires and preferences. But some might argue that this interpretation is too narrow, excluding, as it does, the interest everyone has in not being exploited—in not being treated, as Kant puts it, 'as a means, merely, rather than as an end in itself'. The absence of consent might be thought to be a crucial factor here.

At the time of writing the original article, I wasn't sure whether this latter sort of consideration deserved to be given any weight in this context. Now, however, I am convinced that it does not. Bear in mind that we are talking about an embryo or foetus that is non-viable, and *a fortiori* does not have the potential for acquiring those characteristics that mark off normal human existence from that of lower animals. Now ask yourself whether it would be rational to have such qualms about experimenting on a live but non-viable (and anaesthetized) *non-human* embryo or foetus, at a comparable stage of development. I think almost everyone would reply that it was not rational. But it then follows, I think, that to judge otherwise in the case of the human embryo or foetus would be indefensibly *speciesist*. One would be saying, in effect, that Kant's precept was applicable to one embryo or foetus and nòt to another, solely in virtue of the species to which it belonged. And that, I believe, defies rational justification.

That said, however, there may be all kinds of contingent considerations, some of the 'thin end of the wedge' variety, that weigh in practice against experimenting on live human embryos or foetuses beyond that stage of brain development at which it would be appropriate to judge that human life had begun.

Finally, though, why did I exclude the case in which an embryo or foetus is deliberately kept alive to beyond the point at which human life begins, for the purpose of experimenting on it? My thought here was that death is, other things being equal, a misfortune for an individual and that therefore, by allowing such a being to come into existence, under circumstances in which it cannot ultimately survive, one is responsible for bringing about such a misfortune. (One might argue that, in the circumstances, death is not a misfortune, since the individual has no prospect of worthwhile life anyway. But then *that itself* is, one might say, a misfortune for that individual—a misfortune one has needlessly brought about.) Here too, one must be careful to avoid speciesist traps. But if a given human embryo once had the potential for worthwhile life, then it may be wrong to allow it to develop to the point at which there is a human being who, though no longer viable, could be regarded as having a strong retrospective interest in one's not having allowed that opportunity for worthwhile life to slip away.

2 THE DOCTOR, THE PILL, AND THE FIFTEEN-YEAR-OLD GIRL
A case study in medical ethics and law
IAN KENNEDY

In this article I shall investigate the ethical and legal implications of prescribing oral contraceptives to young girls. This is a matter both of topical interest and of great concern. It is part of a wider debate about the relationship between parents and their children, particularly in their dealings with others. I have chosen to examine it here, however, because, in addition to its intrinsic importance, it is an issue which demonstrates how law and moral philosophy may intersect and interact with medicine.

I hardly need to say that this is an issue on which people have strongly held views. My aim here is to present a scheme for understanding and analysing the problems involved and to explore ways of arriving at answers. Since the answers must be ones we can live with, this will also mean, of course, that I shall have to explore the implications of some of the answers that others advocate.

The hypothetical case I want to consider is as follows. A girl of fifteen approaches her doctor and asks him to prescribe contraceptive pills. The girl, in making her request, makes it clear to the doctor that she does not want her parents to be told that she has consulted him on this matter. The doctor knows that the girl is fifteen years old. The doctor is the family doctor and knows the girl's parents. Finally, the doctor knows that the girl is asking for the pill because she is contemplating having sexual intercourse, rather than for any other medical reason.

Let me quickly add a couple of comments about these assumptions. I have assumed that the doctor knows the girl's family because this is the hard case. The problems are different and, perhaps, easier to solve if the girl has run away from home, or gone to another town and, for example, registered with a GP on a temporary basis. I am also prepared to assume throughout that the doctor tries to persuade the girl to involve her parents but that she adamantly refuses. Finally, you will notice that I say that the girl is contemplating intercourse. I will consider in due course what significance, if any, should be attached to the fact that she has already had, or not already had, intercourse.

The first question that has to be considered before we proceed further is whether, given all the circumstances, the pill would be appropriate treatment for the girl. Treatment, of course, is a concept which has moral and social, as well as technical, dimensions. Merely for a doctor to describe something within his technical competence as 'treatment' does not necessarily make it so. The term 'treatment' connotes something which not only *can* be done, but is also morally and socially warranted. Here, however, the question being asked is whether, simply in medical-technical terms, the pill is appropriate treatment. I will assume for the sake of argument that it is and that there are, for example, no counter-indications or medical-technical reasons which argue against prescription.

A second question then arises. Are there any relevant factors of a non-medical-technical nature which the doctor is obliged to consider before he responds to her request? Can the doctor, having decided that the pill is appropriate, all things being equal, then go ahead and prescribe or refuse to prescribe without further ado? I will return to the issue of refusal at a later stage. I merely point out here that some argue that the doctor is under no obligation to prescribe the pill, and may refuse to do so, since the girl is not ill in the accepted sense. As an alternative, it is suggested that the doctor can impose a condition that the girl agrees to her parents being involved, even when it is clear that she does not want this; so that the condition is tantamount to a refusal. It is by no means clear that these arguments are sound; whether they are or not is something that I shall consider later. But, for the moment, I will assume that the doctor would wish to prescribe the pill.

Rephrasing the question slightly, are there any necessary preliminary conditions which have to be satisfied? Clearly, the answer must be that there are both ethical and legal conditions to be met. I will consider these in turn.

Ethics

The girl has said that she wants the contraceptives; but is this ethically sufficient? Ought the doctor to prescribe them on her say-so, given the assumptions made above? Can the doctor, in other words, rely and act upon this purported exercise of authority by the girl?

Any attempt to answer these questions must be by reference to principles and to the analysis such principles allow. This is the traditional mode of thinking and analysis both in ethics and in law. I suppose that, for me, the relevant starting-point in any ethical analysis must be the principle of respect for persons as persons. What this must mean here is that a doctor has a duty to respect the integrity and individuality of the person (or patient) before him. One, more specific, duty derived from this is the duty to respect the person's autonomy. Respect for autonomy in turn forms a basis for the derivation of further, yet more specific principles, the most important of which, in the present context, is the principle of consent.

It is consent and respect for autonomy that I shall be concentrating on. Here, the girl has purported to act autonomously and has given her consent for the doctor to treat her. (It should be borne in mind that the doctor must, *inter alia*, take the girl's blood pressure, so there will, in legal language, be a *touching* for which consent is needed.) In the language of principles, therefore, the questions can be posed as follows. Must the doctor respect this purported exercise of autonomy? Can he act on the girl's consent?

To pose these questions at all is implicitly to admit that there may be circumstances in which it would be wrong to act on the girl's say-so. She may not, as the expression goes, know her own mind. This gives the clue to what the analysis must focus on. Consent can only be valid (that is, ethically be relied upon) if it is genuinely an expression of autonomy. It will be an expression of autonomy only if the girl is capable of being, or competent to be, autonomous. The girl must be someone who is capable of weighing rationally her decision and its consequences for her and her way of life and values. Notice that this is not the same as saying that she *has* weighed this particular decision, since it is the prerogative of all of us to be irrational. It is an unsolved problem, however, and one to which I shall return, how irrational a person can be and still be judged competent or capable.

This is because capacity is judged by others. In the context of medical care, autonomy is, in effect, a status granted by other people. They have to decide whether paternalism is called for, or whether a person shall be allowed to rule his own life. In our example, the person doing the judging is the doctor. And, clearly, being in a position to make such a judgement vests the doctor with very great power, a power which is virtually beyond regulation or control. For it will be very hard subsequently to challenge whatever decision the doctor may reach, if only because he may insist that, on the facts available to him *at that moment*, his decision was justified. There would normally be no evidence to the contrary, save, of course, for the patient's own account, which can ordinarily be argued away by the doctor as being necessarily partial, the product of illness or perhaps of anger or confusion.

We have argued that consent is derived from autonomy, but that autonomy need be respected only if the person is judged capable. Given how important such a judgement is, in terms of the power it vests in the doctor to grant the patient or deprive him of the right to self-rule, it is clearly of crucial importance to identify the criteria by which capacity is to be judged. Various criteria, or sets of criteria, can be extracted from the literature on consent and capacity. Probably the best recent (1982) discussion is the Report in the United States of the President's Commission for the Study of Ethical and Legal Problems in Medicine and Biomedical and Behavioral Research, entitled *Making Health Care Decisions*.[1] I will consider each proposed criterion in turn.

The 'content' or 'outcome' approach

This view has it that a person's capacity to decide for himself depends upon, and is to be judged by reference to, the content of his decision or the outcome which will follow any particular decision made in purported exercise of autonomy. The effect of this approach is that if the content or outcome is of a particular nature, the person is judged to be lacking capacity, with the consequence that his consent (or refusal of consent) must (not may) ethically be ignored. Of course, everything turns on what content or outcomes are to be taken to be indicative of incapacity. In analysing this question, it ought to be borne in mind that the question of the patient's capacity almost always arises because the doctor or the patient's relatives disagree with the patient's decision. You will not see arguments about capacity when the doctor and relatives, on the one hand, and the patient, on the other, are in full agreement. But merely disagreeing with the content of a decision or not approving the consequences of it cannot by themselves serve as criteria for determining capacity. It may be, of course, that the likely consequences of the decision are so bad, as judged by others, that they cause the doctor to doubt the patient's ability to weigh the various factors involved. But putting the point this way suggests that it is not the particular consequences, or the content, of the decision, but rather the patient's ability to weigh these up for himself, which is being relied upon as the criterion of capacity. I shall return to this point later.

Suffice it to say here that it is a dangerous confusion to regard the outcome or content of a decision as *in itself* a criterion of capacity, as opposed to being merely evidence of the satisfaction of some other criterion. Such an approach purports to respect each person's autonomy. In effect, however, it serves as a blueprint for undermining that autonomy on any occasion when a person with power, in our case a doctor, thinks that the patient's decision is bad or unreasonable. While masquerading as respectful of autonomy, it provides a recipe for substituted judgement (that is, the supplanting of the patient's judgement by that of the doctor) or paternalism. It means that a patient who opts for a decision which is inconsistent with widely held values, or is otherwise unconventional, runs the risk of being labelled as *ipso facto* incapable of knowing his own mind and reaching his own decisions.

The invalidity of this criterion becomes apparent as soon as it is examined thoughtfully. It is perhaps important to remember, therefore, that it is an approach which is very commonly resorted to by all professionals, not only doctors. There is a natural tendency for the doctor and others to believe that they know best, and therefore to think that if a decision on the part of a patient or client seems to them unwise or uncalled for, they need not regard it as binding on them. Unless the patient is correspondingly determined and articulate, the reality of medical practice, as with other client–professional contacts, can be that the outcome test is what the doctor actually acts on. That this is unethical, an abuse of power, has still to enter the thinking of very many doctors.

If the outcome or content approach is invalid, then it cannot be used by our doctor to determine whether the fifteen-year-old girl knows her own mind. Her capacity cannot, therefore, be made to depend on whether the doctor thinks sexual intercourse is something young girls in general, or she in particular, should engage in.

The status approach

The basis of this approach is to argue that a particular status carries with it, by necessary implication, a lack of capacity. A familiar example of this form of argument is the assertion that if someone is mentally ill, he is, by virtue of belonging to the class of mentally ill people and having the corresponding status, incapable of arriving at considered decisions which may properly be relied upon. Another, equally familiar, example is the status of minority. Leaving aside for a moment the question of what constitutes minority, the view is that, by being a minor, a person *ipso facto* lacks capacity.

The invalidity of this approach is equally obvious. Merely to belong to a given class does not entail incapacity, except and unless that class is defined by reference to lack of capacity. The question to be asked, therefore, is whether all mentally ill persons or minors must, once they are so categorized, be considered to be incapable of making autonomous decisions on any matter, at any time. Unless the answer is 'Yes', it will be clear that the class is not defined in terms of capacity, but by other factors with, at best, a merely contingent connection with capacity, such as symptoms of illness or number of birthdays. Clearly, someone may be mentally ill, or only fifteen years old, and yet still have the capacity to decide and act autonomously. The mental illness may only affect certain aspects of behaviour or feeling or thought, or may coexist with periods of lucidity. The fifteen-year-old's decision not to go to the cinema with her parents, for example, or to go to her school counsellor for advice, would be regarded as properly for her to make.

The fundamental flaw in the status approach is that it takes no account of the individuality of each person. Respect for autonomy, however, involves respect for each person's individuality. It demands, therefore, that any criterion intended to determine when someone is incapable of being autonomous should, equally, be respectful of that person's individuality. The test must look at, and be sensitive to, the qualities of the individual. Merely placing him in a class is far too gross a test of capacity. It denies respect to the individual as an individual, and must therefore be rejected.

There is a further, supplementary, objection to the status approach. Minority as a status is usually associated with being below a certain fixed age, whether it be sixteen, eighteen, or twenty-one. While it is clearly necessary, for legal purposes, to choose a definite age, even though it is bound to some extent to be arbitrary, there is no such necessity in the case of ethical analysis. Ethics need take account only of the fact that there is such a thing as minority, that there is, for every individual, a stage of development at which that individual is immature. This immediately makes it clear that it is, in fact, maturity that is the criterion, rather than minority. And since maturation is a process that will necessarily vary from individual to individual, the adoption of one particular age or date as the benchmark of maturity in all persons is clearly untenable. Indeed, even the law, which must, for the sake of certainty, adopt some fixed point of reference for minority, defines it differently for different purposes. For example, the age of consent for the purposes of volunteering for the armed services is not the same as the age at which someone may vote. Equally, the age at which a person may marry without parental consent is not the same as the age at which the same person may consent to sexual intercourse.

As regards consent to medical treatment, the picture is sometimes muddied by those who argue, first, that the *law* requires the consent of parent(s), or of someone *in loco parentis*, before a doctor may treat someone under sixteen years of age, and, secondly, that since it is ordinarily morally obligatory to uphold the law, it is therefore *ethically* wrong for a doctor to treat someone under sixteen, save in an emergency, in the absence of parental consent (or some legally acceptable substitute). Now I concede that ordinarily one ought to obey the law. But it is as well to get the law straight! It is not the law, nor in my view has it ever been, that a doctor may not treat a person under sixteen without another's authority. I shall be arguing this point more fully later on, when I come to examine the law. Suffice it to say now that once the legal argument is shown to be spurious, the ethical argument built on it, that sixteen is the magic age for consent, can safely be ignored. (But see now the Postscript, p. 64.)

It follows, then, that in our case the fact that the girl asking for the pill is only fifteen years old cannot ethically be regarded as settling the question whether she has the capacity to act autonomously. Evidence it may be; but evidence of maturity, or lack thereof, since maturity is the key.

The individual's capacity to comprehend

It should be clear from what has been said so far that the only valid criterion of capacity is the ability of the particular individual to comprehend the nature and consequences of the proposed procedure. This is a test which is specific to each individual and is thereby aimed at maximizing respect for each person's autonomy. It makes maturity the crucial determinant, the maturity that consists in having a stable set of values and outlook on life and the ability to weigh the proposed procedure in the light of these so as to arrive at a considered decision. As a criterion it differs from the outcome or content approach in that the content of the decision has to conform to the girl's set of values rather than those of her doctor or some other allegedly objective scale. It is the approach that the President's Commission refers to as the 'functional approach', because it 'focuses on an individual's actual functioning in decision-making situations'.[2]

If, however, it is suggested that capacity must not be measured by reference to whether any decision is reasonable, or objectively acceptable, the objection may be made that such a criterion errs too much on the side of subjectivity. By so doing it may, in effect, reduce the autonomy of the girl. This would be so, if it meant that a decision which, by any account, would entail harm for the girl, was to be respected because it accorded with her world-view or scheme of values. Acting on this decision, it is said, may not further the girl's autonomy, since, if it flows from ill-considered premises or a skewed perception of the world, it could mean that she exposes herself to avoidable and irreparable harm, and thereby reduces her ability to enjoy autonomy in the future.

There is obviously some force to this argument. It is as valid here as it is in the case of the mentally ill person whose decision is the product of a very strange perception of the world. But there is, equally, force in the counter-argument that this could usher in through the back door what has already been refused formal admittance, namely the outcome or content approach. Clearly, we are not far from the content approach if we say that the girl's present decision should be overridden because it is unreasonable, or may have dangerous consequences. One should bear in mind the power vested in the doctor, in that it is he who is the arbiter of capacity, and also that it is he who is likely to wish most strongly that the girl would opt for a course other than the one she has in fact chosen. Given this, we can see that the doctor may well pay lip service to the test of her ability to comprehend the procedure proposed, and yet judge her incapable by virtue of the decision she arrives at. Of course, this would be done for what the doctor, at least, would regard as the best possible motives. It would, for all that, be strongly paternalistic. It would also mean that the proposed criterion of capacity is, in the event, unworkable, since it provides insufficient safeguards for the individual. As the President's Commission put it,

The fact that a patient belongs to a category of people who are often unable to make general decisions for their own well-being or that an individual makes a highly idiosyncratic decision should alert health professionals to the greater possibility of decisional incapacity. But it does not conclusively resolve the matter.[3]

Thus, something more must be added to this criterion. The first additional factor must be that, in enquiring whether the girl before him comprehends the nature and consequences of the procedure proposed, the doctor must act with total integrity. He must recognize and accept the reason for the enquiry, namely the obligation to respect the girl's autonomy, and must devote an appropriate amount of time and care to pursuing it. He must use language which is comprehensible, and must be conscious of the power disequilibrium, which is a feature of virtually all doctor–patient relationships.

The second thing that needs to be added is that any enquiry into capacity must take account of certain presumptions. The President's Commission recommends that if a minor patient is over fourteen it should be presumed that she is capable of deciding for herself, so that evidence would have to be adduced to rebut the presumption. In practical terms, this would mean that the doctor would have to note carefully and be prepared to stand by whatever evidence persuaded him that a girl over fourteen lacked capacity. Such a presumption would not decide the issue of capacity, but would provide the starting-point of an enquiry about whether it can be rebutted on the strength of the facts in the particular case.

I find the Commission's recommendation attractive, in respect of its use of this notion of presumptions. The difficulty, however, lies in the way it rejects status, in the form of under or over sixteen, only to readopt an age criterion later, in the form of under or over fourteen. The difference, it will be said, lies in the fact that the first criterion is arbitrary and inflexible, the second flexible and merely the first stage in a necessary enquiry. Accepting this, it is none the less arguable that, in practice, there is a danger of the one age simply supplanting the other as a hard and fast cut-off point. On balance, this may be a necessary risk that proponents of the criterion must run. Ultimately, they can only place their faith in the doctor's integrity and hope that the presumptions will operate as intended.

The final element that should be incorporated into this criterion, to make it as sensitive as possible to the principle of respect for autonomy, is some sort of device that will maximize the chances of the doctor actually pursuing the necessary enquiry into capacity. What I have in mind is some sort of formalized testing device which would be available to doctors and of which they would be instructed to make use. Such a suggestion is made by the President's Commission, which recommends the adoption of a standardized test, appropriately designed to measure capacity. The Commission refers to this (p. 172, fn. 8) as the 'mental status examination':

The 'mental status examination' is perhaps the best example of how professional expertise can be enlisted in making assessments of incapacity. Such an evaluation is intended, among other things, to elicit the patient's orientation to person, place, time, and situation, the patient's mood and affect, and the content of thought and perception, with an eye to any delusions and hallucinations; to assess intellectual capacity, that is, the patient's ability to comprehend abstract ideas and to make a reasoned judgment based on that ability; to review past history for evidence of any psychiatric disturbance that might affect the patient's current judgment; and to test the patient's recent and remote memory and logical sequencing.

This sort of test would have the merit of emphasizing that judgements of capacity are not really medical-technical but rather matters of common sense. A test designed by those having some knowledge of maturity could, then, ensure that the question of capacity was not left to be decided entirely by the doctor's own, possibly idiosyncratic, judgement. This is not to say that such a procedural device would supplant the exercise, by the doctor, of his own judgement. But it might serve to constrain it within limits set by others.

If this criterion of capacity, the ability to comprehend the nature and consequences of the proposed procedure, is accepted, subject to the suggested provisos, it means that the fifteen-year-old girl can give valid consent to the prescription of the pill, provided she meets the criterion. The doctor, therefore, once satisfied of this, is entitled to prescribe the pill as a matter of good medical ethics. The fact that she is fifteen years old would, all other things being equal, be neither here nor there. As to whether she does meet the necessary criterion of maturity, it could be said that the very act of consulting a doctor to get contraceptives is an act of maturity. It would then be for the doctor to put before the girl the various disadvantages involved in her decision (assuming her to be aware of the advantages). Notice that it is for the doctor to do so. It is not open to him to object that she is incapable of deciding because she is ignorant of the relevant implications. Once a relationship of doctor and patient is created between them, it is the doctor's duty to place before her that information which will allow her to reach an informed and considered decision.

Other considerations

At this point, it may be objected that all the emphasis has been on respect for autonomy and that I have ignored at least two other relevant considerations. They are the claim of the parents to be involved in the decision, and the need to consider the interests of the family and the possible effect on the family of a decision to prescribe. I will consider these in turn.

THE PARENTS' CLAIM

The parents' claim to be informed by the doctor, if their daughter should seek contraceptives, is often presented in an unattractive form, as if it were really a property issue. 'She is our daughter. Therefore we have a right to be consulted.' This is how it is often put. Clearly, it is not, when properly formulated, a property claim. Rather, it is an assertion that, since the parents have responsibilities towards their daughter, so they are entitled to be consulted and to be involved in her decisions. But does this latter proposition flow from the former? In the recent case of *Gillick* v. *West Norfolk and Wisbech Area Health Authority*,[4] in which these issues were aired, Mrs Gillick argued that she had rights in respect of her children by virtue of being their parent and custodian. What are these rights? They are, I submit, only those rights necessary to perform parental obligations. A parent is, in my view, the trustee of the interests of the child. This being so, the primary obligation of the parent is to bring the child to an enjoyment of autonomy, as free as possible from constraints on this enjoyment. In short, parental obligations are to be understood as being primarily autonomy-enhancing. This means that the parent has an obligation initially to protect the child, while she is still immature, and thereafter, as the child acquires maturity, to leave her to make her own decisions and her own mistakes.

If this is correct and the girl is, on the criterion proposed above, judged to be capable of making her own decisions, there would seem to be no justification for the parent insisting, as did Mrs Gillick, on being informed and consulted until her daughter reaches the age of sixteen. As we have seen, the age of the girl does not suffice to determine her capacity to make decisions.

Someone might retort that it is a crime for a man to engage in sexual intercourse with a girl under sixteen years of age and that, once supplied with contraceptives, the fifteen-year-old girl may, by engaging in intercourse, become a party to a crime. The fact that it is a crime, however, does not mean that the parents are entitled to be consulted in circumstances where it is conceded that the girl is autonomous. As I shall argue later, I believe that the doctor is under a legal obligation to treat the girl, assuming her to be autonomous. That a male partner may subsequently commit a crime would, presumably, be a matter of regret for the doctor, but it is not necessarily a reason for forsaking his commitment to her autonomy or his pledge of confidentiality.

This is not to say that the parents have no claim at all. It is to suggest only that their claim may not weigh heaviest in the scale. A doctor may wish to involve the girl's parents. Indeed, the girl herself may wish to do so, but be deterred by her belief that they would not understand. In such circumstances the girl's claim, assuming her to have been judged capable of making her own decisions, is, I submit, to be preferred to that of the parents. To argue otherwise involves saying one or other of two things, neither of which can be seriously sustained. The first is that proposed by Mrs Gillick that, until her daughter reaches sixteen, she has a right to be consulted (and presumably a right of veto) over *any* decision her daughter may make concerning medical treatment. Such a conclusion falls foul of the objections to the status approach outlined earlier. Taken to its extreme, it implies that, on the girl's sixteenth birthday, some magical process takes place whereby maturity and the capacity to make decisions are suddenly visited upon her. It ignores all the arguments concerning the process of gaining maturity.

Alternatively, one would have to argue that, despite being capable of making her own decisions (as I am assuming that she is) the girl is somehow unable to act responsibly, and that her parents must, for that reason, be consulted. This is clearly contradictory. If autonomy is self-enhancing then I submit that the girl's autonomy is to be preferred for at least three reasons. First, pregnancy, which is a likely consequence of her failing to obtain contraceptives, can hardly be described as self-enhancing in these circumstances. Secondly, denying the girl the right to act autonomously, when it is granted that she is capable of doing so, is clearly autonomy-reducing. Thirdly, exercise of the power to make her own decisions is, by contrast, autonomy-enhancing and consequently to be preferred.

THE INTERESTS OF THE FAMILY

The second consideration which it may be said I have overlooked is the interests of the family. Here I assume that the doctor, being the family doctor also, would wish to take account of the interests of the family, considered as a unit. He may decide that the girl's wishes are in conflict with the best interests of the family as a family. This could persuade him not to accede to the girl's request, even though he accepted that she was capable of making her own decisions.

There are several obvious objections to giving greater weight to the claims of the family than to the principle of respect for autonomy. The first is that there is no reason to think that the doctor is the best judge, or indeed any judge, of where the family's true interests lie. The doctor may, for example, decide on a given course of conduct because it seems to him to be the best way of keeping the family together. But the underlying assumption may be invalid. Maybe it would be better for this particular family to break up. And whether it should break up or not is, surely, a matter exclusively for members of that family to decide, unless or until others, perhaps including the doctor, are consulted. For the doctor to interfere, unasked, on the basis of limited information and irrelevant personal preference is wholly un-warranted.

The second objection is that the family includes the daughter. Thus, the family's interests must include her interests. Where her views do not, or may not, coincide with those of other members of the family, it is a false antithesis to contrast her views with the interests of the family. It is a case, rather, of there being a division of opinion within the family. In such circumstances there is no obvious reason why the doctor should prefer the views (or what he imagines to be the views) of other members of the family to those of the girl. The only argument that one could advance is, assuming the doctor's views of what the rest of the family wanted to be correct, that they knew best. But if it has already been granted that the girl is capable of acting autonomously, such an argument must fail, unless it means that they know best who agree with the doctor. And to say that is to substitute the exercise of power for respect for principled analysis.

The final objection to preferring the alleged interests of the family is a more pragmatic one. The girl, in approaching the doctor, has stipulated that he may not consult or involve her parents. This is at least *prima facie* evidence that the family is not an integrated unit with a common set of interests which can be identified and served. If the doctor persists in thinking that it is, the major casualty will be the girl herself, who will lose faith in her doctor, or seek help elsewhere, or even abandon efforts to get help from any doctor.

This concludes my discussion of capacity. If the girl, on proper enquiry by the doctor, is found to understand the nature and consequences of taking the pill, including, obviously, its risks, then she must be judged capable of making her own decisions and the doctor may act on her request. It only remains to say that if the doctor decides, on the criterion I have proposed, that the girl is not capable of making her own decisions, then he may not treat her on her say-so alone. Ethically speaking, he is bound to ignore her consent. Doing so is entirely in keeping with the principle of respect for autonomy, since it is autonomy-enhancing to protect the immature from their ill-considered decisions. It is also in conformity with the principle of beneficence, in that the doctor is, under the circumstances, acting for the girl's own good and to protect her from harm.

CONFIDENTIALITY

Let me turn now to a separate ethical issue raised by the girl's request that her parents not be informed that she is asking for contraceptive pills. The question can be simply put. Is the doctor, if he proceeds to prescribe the pills, ethically entitled thereafter to inform the parents despite the girl's request to the contrary?

It may well be that the doctor should try to persuade the girl to involve her parents. In so doing, the doctor pays proper heed to the interests of the parents and the family and also gives the girl the opportunity to reflect further on her decision. In some cases the girl may change her mind, persuaded, for example, that her parents may be more understanding than she supposed. In our case, however, she remains unmoved.

One principle derived from the general obligation of respect for each person is that of respect for promises. An essential feature of respect for another is honouring his trust, and keeping promises is one example of observing this trust. Implicit in the doctor–patient relationship is the promise that information imparted to the doctor *qua* doctor will not be divulged. There are, obviously, good pragmatic, as well as principled, reasons for this, since the patient will not otherwise confide in his doctor and the doctor will be unable to do his job. Thus, without the need for it to be made explicit, the doctor is obliged to keep his patient's confidences. It follows, *a fortiori*, that he is obliged to do so if the patient explicitly demands it, as in our case, where the girl makes it a condition of the relationship.

There are those, however, who argue that, despite obligations of confidence, the doctor is entitled, or even obliged, to tell the parents. Can there be any justification for this, if the girl forbids it and it is conceded that she is capable of acting autonomously? The only argument one could give is that the parents have an interest in knowing and that this interest transcends any duty the doctor might have towards the girl. But the first difficulty with this argument is that, if this is what the doctor believes, he is under an obligation to make it clear at the outset of the consultation that he cannot agree to the girl's conditions. This would give the girl the opportunity to end the consultation and go elsewhere. But there may be nowhere else that it is feasible for her to go, or else the mere fact of discussing the issue, before going elsewhere, may have alerted the doctor to what the girl is contemplating.

Further difficulties in the argument that the parents have a right to know then appear. The doctor may prefer the interests of the parents because of what he assumes (or knows) them to want. Alternatively, he may do so out of respect for the principle of beneficence. I shall take the latter point first. For the doctor to assume that he knows what is best for the girl would, I submit, be an unwarranted act of strong paternalism, whereby the doctor merely substitutes his judgement for hers. If it is granted that the girl knows her own mind, then the presumption must be that she knows what is best for herself. The fact that the doctor happens to disagree with her is not a sufficient reason for him to ignore or override her wishes, or if it is, it gives rise to the general principle that the doctor should always be the final arbiter of the best interests of his patient. This principle has only to be stated to be seen to be unacceptable; it would be unhesitatingly rejected by patients and doctors alike. Clearly, it has no place in sound medical ethics.

As regards the first point, there are powerful pragmatic, as well as principled, reasons why the doctor should not prefer the presumed interests of the parents. It would mean that any trust between the girl and the doctor would be destroyed, possibly for ever. It might even lead to a loss of confidence in doctors in general, with consequent risks to the girl's future health and well-being. Moreover, if it became generally known that it was considered ethically acceptable for doctors to inform on girls to their parents, girls in the future might be deterred altogether from consulting doctors to get contraceptive advice or treatment, with all that this could entail.

For all these reasons, therefore, I submit that there is no good case for the doctor to breach the girl's confidence and inform her parents.

Law

As with many other aspects of the relationship between a doctor and his patients, it is not only ethics that would seek to regulate the prescription of contraceptives to the fifteen-year-old. The law is also involved. Some argue rather forlornly that the law has no place in the practice of medicine. It is, they say, far too blunt an instrument to deal sensitively with the complexities of the doctor–patient relationship. The answer, of course, is that there is nothing intrinsically to distinguish the relationship between a doctor and his patient from that of any other professional and his client. Moreover, there are things that the doctor is allowed by law to do, which others are not, and this privilege must be the object of proper regulation and scrutiny. And if some of those things that the doctor may do to another involve conduct that society takes very seriously, for example touching, cutting, and restraining, then clearly the regulation and scrutiny must take the form of law.

It is one thing to say that the law is involved. Unfortunately, it is quite another thing to say precisely what the law requires. The reasons for this are not hard to understand. For example, new procedures and technology have posed new problems for which the law, looking backwards for guidance as it inevitably does, has no immediate answers. Also, there has been a growing tendency, in the past few years, for issues to be tested in the courts, either because of a lack of confidence in other less formal methods of resolution or because of a desire to clarify the respective rights and duties of the parties involved. Such litigation does not always serve to clarify the law. Frequently the resolution of an issue before the courts serves rather to bring into sharper focus the unsolved legal questions that remain; indeed, it may itself prompt such questions. And, of course, such a legal minefield is a heaven-sent opportunity for commentators and academics confidently to map the ways out (all different!), knowing that they will not have to leave the safety of their own rooms. If anyone is to be blown up, metaphorically speaking, it will be the doctor or the patient. It will come as no surprise to discover that doctors cannot, generally speaking, muster the same *sang froid*. They have to get their hands dirty in their day-to-day practice and, if there is to be law, it should, they protest, at least give them clear guidance as to what is permissible.

The complaint seems entirely just. But, sadly, there are relatively few ways, within the English system, of making the law clear. Parliament appears to be unwilling to provide any leadership in clarifying medico-legal issues, important though they are. The only other law-makers are the courts and they depend on having a case brought before them, a case, moreover, the facts of which are such as to allow the laying down of rules of more general applicability. The fundamental drawback of relying on the courts, apart from the interstitial nature of the process (*ad hoc* and random, filling in gaps as they are encountered), is its unfairness. It would ordinarily involve suing a doctor or putting one in the dock so as to test the lawfulness of what he has done. It cannot be right that society's method of developing its medical law should be at the expense of some doctor, who up till then may well have thought, and indeed been assured, that he was acting lawfully.

There is one other role that the courts could play, that of making declaratory judgements. A declaratory judgement is one in which the court is invited to say what the law would be if someone decided to embark on a particular course of conduct. It is a device commonly employed in the United States, where courts have, for example, been asked to rule whether it would be lawful for a doctor, under certain specified circumstances, to discontinue certain forms of life-sustaining treatment. The attraction of this procedure notwithstanding, the English courts have been slow to adopt it, being reluctant to solve hypothetical disputes, as opposed to real ones.

What has been true of law-makers has been true equally of law-reformers. The Law Commission has studiously avoided all contact with medical law. The various Royal Colleges have taken their professional preference for self-regulation to the point at which they have often tended to oppose any proposed reform of the law, even where its aim is clarification for the benefit of their members. All in all, it is a rather sorry state of affairs; a vacuum in legal leadership. The contrast with Australia and Canada, with their energetic and helpful Law Reform Commissions, and with the United States and its President's Commission (now admittedly defunct) is a depressing one.

There is no alternative, therefore, but for me to try to take to heart my own strictures against academics and offer an analysis of what, in my view, the law currently provides on the issue of prescription of contraceptive pills to fifteen-year-old girls.

It would be comforting if the law were seen to reflect what I have already argued to be good medical ethics. As will become clear, however, things may not be quite that simple. I take as a point of reference, throughout my analysis, the judgement of Woolf J. in *Gillick* v. *West Norfolk and Wisbech A.H.A.*[5] Mrs Gillick brought an action against the local Area Health Authority. She sought a declaration from the court that a Health Service Notice (HN (80) 46), issued by the Department of Health and Social Security in December 1980, had no authority in law. The Health Service Notice in question outlined arrangements for the organiz-ation and development of NHS family planning services. It was accompanied by a memorandum of guidance which, in its revised version, suggested that a doctor was entitled, albeit only in exceptional circumstances, to prescribe contraceptives to a girl under sixteen without consulting her parents.

There were what Woolf J. called 'two principal limbs'[6] to Mrs Gillick's case. The first was that the Notice and accompanying memorandum advises doctors, in effect, to commit a crime, as being accessories to unlawful sexual intercourse with a girl under sixteen, contrary to section 6 of the Sexual Offences Act, 1956. Notice that the offender under section 6 is the male partner who has sexual intercourse. The section is intended to protect young girls. They are considered to be the victims of the offence and cannot themselves be held guilty of any offence. The doctor, therefore, would have to be the accessory of the male partner.

The second limb of the case was that, in authorizing doctors to give advice and treatment to girls under sixteen years of age, without their parents' consent, the guidance, if it did not advocate a criminal offence, was nevertheless inconsistent with the rights of parents over their children. For our purposes, this can be reduced to the proposition that a girl under sixteen may not in law give a valid consent to treatment (save, perhaps, in certain cases of emergency).

Consent to treatment

This second argument is the more easily answered and I shall therefore deal with it first. Woolf J. found it 'most surprising that there is no previous authority of the courts of this country whether a child under 16 can consent to medical treatment'. His conclusion, however, was in line with the analysis I offered earlier and, therefore, suggests that on this issue ethics and law coincide. He declared,

The fact that a child is under the age of 16 does not mean automatically that she cannot give consent to any treatment. Whether or not a child is capable of giving the necessary consent will depend on the child's maturity and understanding and the nature of the consent which is required. The child must be capable of making a reasonable assessment of the advantages and disadvantages of the treatment proposed, so the consent if given can be properly and fairly described as a true consent.[7]

Woolf J. referred to the fact that the Health Service Notice specifically states that it 'would be most unusual to provide advice about or methods of contraception without parental consent'. This indeed is a salient feature of the Notice, that it says this should be done only in exceptional circumstances. Woolf J. went on to say, however, that 'in the exceptional case there remains a discretion for the clinical judgement of the doctor whether or not to prescribe contraception'.[8] The supposed parental right to be involved in the treatment and care of a child under sixteen, regardless of that child's level of maturity, was, therefore, rejected by the court. All that the court was prepared to concede was that the doctor should try to persuade the child to involve her parents and that the capacity (or, in legal terms, the competence) of the child varied with her understanding and maturity, and the seriousness of the procedure involved. Thus, Woolf J. was prepared to suggest that 'it is unlikely that a child under the age of 16 will ever be regarded by the courts as being capable of giving consent to sterilisation'.[9]

One final point ought to be made. Once the child is over sixteen, then, in law at least, she is *prima facie* competent to give consent, by virtue of section 8(1) of the Family Law Reform Act, 1969. The doctor is still, of course, ethically and legally obliged to ensure that the sixteen-year-old before him is *actually* capable of making her own decisions.

Accessory to crime

I turn now to the other legal issue, the question of whether the doctor, in prescribing the contraceptive pills, is an accessory to a crime. If he were to be so judged, all the previous analysis would be irrelevant. It would be of no consequence that the girl was capable and competent to consent and that the doctor could rely on her consent without reference to the parents. Much, therefore, hangs on the answer to be arrived at. If Mrs Gillick were successful in this argument, she would achieve her objective, albeit by what, from her point of view, was a less satisfactory route, since it would not depend on parental rights. Indeed, if the courts were to find that the doctor would be guilty of a crime, the question of parental consent would be irrelevant. For, if it were a crime, the fact that the parents had consented to their daughter's being treated would be neither here nor there, since they may not waive the operation of the criminal law. This rather obvious point seems to have been lost on Mrs Gillick's legal advisers, since the form of declaratory relief they sought included both the proposition that no child under sixteen should be treated without parental consent, and the somewhat contradictory proposition that, if the doctor were to treat any girl under sixteen, he would be guilty as an accessory.

In law, a person is liable as an accessory if he aids, abets, counsels, or procures the commission of a crime. On some occasions, a person may be charged with engaging in only one of these forms of behaviour; on others he may be charged in what Professor Williams calls 'the blunderbuss' way,[10] which includes all of them. It has sometimes been considered correct law to combine aiding with abetting and regard these as committed by an accessory who is present at the scene of a crime, whereas counselling and procuring are combined to describe an accessory who is not present. Smith and Hogan, the leading commentators on criminal law,[11] suggest that such an approach may not always be appropriate and that, in any event, although these words mean different things, 'all four words may be used together to charge a person . . . So long as the evidence establishes that D's [the accused's] conduct satisfied one of the words, that is enough.'[12] Professor Williams comments: 'Any one of the four verbs may be charged, or all four may be charged together (with the conjunctive 'and') and in the same count [of the indictment]. Charging all four is the safest thing to do, because the shades of difference between them are far from clear.'[13]

I propose, therefore, to take each of these words in turn and consider whether the doctor's prescription of contraceptives falls within the meaning of any of them. If it does, then he will be guilty of a crime. In seeking to identify the meaning of these words, it must be remembered that they are legal terms. This means that they will, for the most part, carry their ordinary meaning but that there is also some accretion of technical usage, since they are used in the context of a system which has its own rules. I might add that I will confine myself to that legal analysis which is necessary to solve the problems before us. There are, not surprisingly, a host of subsidiary issues which serve to tempt the analyst but I will endeavour to resist the temptation to become embroiled with them.

I begin with the word 'procure'. According to Lord Widgery CJ in *Attorney General's Reference (No. 1 of 1975)*, 'to procure means to produce by endeavour'. What this means is that there must be 'a causal link between what you do and the commission of the offence'.[14] 'Procure' does not, however, connote any agreement or consensus between the parties. The *Attorney General's Reference* case provides an example, where a man who claimed that he had 'laced' his friend's drinks without the friend's knowledge was found guilty of procuring the offence by his friend of driving with an excess of alcohol in his blood.

Next, there are the words 'abet' and 'counsel'. I take these together since they have a common core of meaning. This is that a person is guilty if he encourages another to commit a crime, or incites him or instigates the crime. There must, in other words, be a consensus between the abettor or counsellor and the perpetrator of the crime. There need not, however, be any causative link between the encouragement and the crime. The encouragement must be operative on the mind of the offender. But it does not have to be the reason why the crime was committed; it may well be that the offender would have committed it anyway.

Finally, there is the word 'aid'. This has its natural meaning of giving help or support, or assisting. Lord Simon in *Lynch* v. *D.P.P. for Northern Ireland*[15] identified the *actus reus* of aiding as 'the supplying of an instrument for a crime or anything essential for its commission'.[16] As will become clear, these words are very important. The *mens rea* of aiding was identified by Devlin J. in *National Coal Board* v. *Gamble*[17] as being the 'intention to aid as well as knowledge of the circumstances',[18] that is, the circumstances which amount to the crime. Devlin's view was cited with approval by Lord Simon in *Lynch*'s case.

A number of propositions can be derived from this definition. The first is that motive must be distinguished from intention. To establish liability as an aider, one need not show that the accused desired the end result. Secondly, there is no need to show encouragement by the aider or any consensus between him and the perpetrator of the crime. Thirdly, the definition establishes that it is not necessary to show that the aider, by his assistance, caused the perpetrator to commit the crime. The aider could, indeed, be guilty even if the perpetrator would have committed the crime in any event. Finally, it may be of help to point out that the cases in which someone is found guilty of aiding usually involve his having helped in such matters as how to commit the crime, for example by supplying a plan of a bank, or what to do it with, for example by providing the means of breaking into a safe, or how to commit the crime more easily (the combination of the safe), or more safely (keeping a look out), or finally, how to get away (driving the get-away car).

It is clear from this analysis of what counts as an accessory, that the doctor *could* be guilty as an accessory. If he prescribes the contraceptive pills with the intention thereby of encouraging the girl to have sexual intercourse, then he will obviously be guilty as an abettor or counsellor. This will be so whether he sees the girl alone or sees her with her male partner. And if the doctor does see both of them he could also be guilty of the crime of conspiracy and possibly of incitement. To be guilty of conspiracy the doctor must have acted 'in pursuance of a criminal purpose held in common'[19] between him and the male partner. He cannot be guilty of conspiracy if he only sees the girl, since he cannot, by section 2(2) of the Criminal Law Act, 1977, conspire with her, as she is the intended victim of the crime. To be guilty of incitement, the doctor must not only intend that the crime be committed but also use some persuasion or pressure in an effort to bring it about.

It will, presumably, be very rare, however, for a doctor to encourage a young girl to engage in sexual intercourse. It will be even rarer for him to incite or conspire with her male partner to do so. To say that a doctor may be guilty of a crime as an accessory by abetting or counselling is to be analytically accurate but somewhat other-worldly. Ordinarily a doctor will not encourage sexual intercourse. Indeed, he will probably seek to discourage it in one so young.

What is quite certain is that the doctor will not be guilty of abetting or counselling if he follows the spirit of the memorandum of guidance issued with the Health Service Notice, which was the object of Mrs Gillick's displeasure. For he will, in that case, have gone through a process of discussion with the girl, will have assessed the situation and explained to her the unwisdom of sexual intercourse at her age. Then, and only then, will he have reached the conclusion that she is one of the 'exceptional cases' envisaged in the Notice, where professional counselling and the prescription of contraceptive pills may be called for, a conclusion that the doctor is likely to have arrived at with regret. In such circumstances, it cannot be argued that the doctor is guilty of encouraging, that is, abetting or counselling.

Equally, given the established meaning of 'procuring', it is hard to see how the doctor can ever be guilty, as an accessory, of procuring unlawful sexual intercourse. He cannot be said to have produced the intercourse by his endeavour. For his prescription of the contraceptive pills is not the cause, the *sine qua non*, of the unlawful intercourse. The male partner can have intercourse with the girl regardless of whether she has been to her doctor or not. Moreover, a charge of procuring would fail on proof that the couple planned to have sexual intercourse in any event, with or without contraceptives. Even if it could be shown that the girl told the doctor that she would not have intercourse if he did not prescribe contraceptives, this would still not be procuring. It might, however, be encouraging, because, in such circumstances, whatever the doctor may have said, it could be argued that, by the very act of prescribing contraceptives, he was encouraging the girl to have intercourse, and was therefore an accessory. Encouraging, however, requires more than the mere provision of assistance or advice. There must also be an *intention to encourage*, and it may be that the doctor could still escape liability on this ground.

The conclusion, therefore, is that, setting aside the obviously very rare case in which a doctor encourages a girl or couple to engage in unlawful sexual intercourse, he does not, by prescribing contraceptive pills, abet, counsel, or procure an offence.

The doctor is thus free to prescribe unless it can be shown that he *aids* in the commission of the offence of unlawful sexual intercourse. The exasperated non-lawyer, having seen the other words defined away, may insist that of course the doctor was guilty of aiding: the other words may have technical meanings, but surely everyone would accept that the doctor lent assistance to the male partner. The doctor knows why the girl wants the pill and that, if he prescribes, the chances are that she will have sexual intercourse. Knowing this, as he must, whether he tries to encourage or discourage the girl is irrelevant. His prescription serves as a green light to further intercourse, removing as it does whatever inhibitions the girl or her male partner may have had as a result of their fear of impregnation. Surely, therefore, the doctor must be guilty of aiding and, as such, be an accessory.

You may recall my saying earlier that words such as 'aid' should, as far as possible, carry their ordinary meaning. But you may also recall my pointing out that words are subject to interpretation by the courts and that, within the legal system, each interpretation serves as a precedent. It is part of the tradition of the legal system that precedents are followed, or treated with great respect, as carrying authority. An obvious reason for this is the certainty and predictability it engenders. Citizens are thereby enabled to know where they stand; they can order their lives confident that they understand what the rules mean. There may be the occasional novel interpretation and new line of precedent but, by and large, certainty is cultivated. The very fact, however, that the law uses words as its tools means that there is a certain inherent uncertainty, or flexibility at least, in meaning. In one way this is a good thing. For it allows the law to develop and change in response to new, or newly perceived, needs. In the criminal law, however, in contrast, say, to commercial law, certainty is regarded as the more important goal, even if secured at the cost of inflexibility. Reasons for this are not hard to find. The most obvious one, perhaps, is the fact that liberty is at stake. Every citizen, one might say, is entitled to know the proper limits of permissible conduct *before* he acts, if the consequence of over-stepping them may be loss of liberty.

With this in mind, it is for you to judge, in the light of the considerations I am about to raise, whether it would be desirable to capture the doctor's conduct under the word 'aid'. Let me begin by saying that the ordinary legal meaning of the word would, in my view, at present exclude the doctor's prescription of contraceptive pills. He would not be an accessory, since the prescription does not amount to 'the supplying of an instrument for a crime or anything essential for its commission'.[20]

If you would wish to see the doctor regarded as guilty, in law, as an accessory, then you will have to reflect on the consequences of defining 'aiding' in such a way as to achieve this. You could well be embarrassed by the precedent it would create. Other conduct, which you would not wish to categorize as criminal, may turn out to be indistinguishable, in this respect, from the doctor's conduct and may therefore leave the actors open to prosecution. In the past, as I have said, aiding has been confined to such matters as how to do the crime, what to do it with, how to do it more safely or easily, and how to get away. And when I say 'more safely', actual cases have been concerned with helping the perpetrator(s) avoid detection. The doctor's conduct fits none of these categories. Before deciding to extend the meaning of 'aid' so as to make him guilty as an accessory, consider the following examples.

A college tutor is visited by one of his students, who says that he is one of a group of students who periodically climb spires in the University to put up flags in support of rag week. Inevitably, in the course of the climb, the stonework of some of the spires is slightly chipped, and sometimes lightning conductors are damaged. (This would amount to criminal damage, under the Criminal Damage Act, 1971). The tutor tells the student that it is an extremely silly thing to do and advises him not to do it (thus not encouraging the student). 'But', the tutor goes on, 'if you insist on climbing spires, for Heaven's sake wear this crash helmet.'

Secondly, suppose that a college tutor is told by one of his rugby-playing students that he intends to settle off the field an old score, arising out of an incident on the field when he was fouled by an opposing player. Again, the tutor points out the folly of such behaviour and the demeaning nature of brawling. But the student insists that he will have his fight. The tutor then says 'I think you are a damned fool, but it might help if you wear these' and hands him some shin guards.

There are, of course, many other examples one could cite. I have chosen these two, as the tutor has some sort of special responsibility for the student and is thus in a position somewhat analogous to that of the doctor. The examples both have to do with mitigating any harm which may come to the student, if he insists on doing what he says, in a context in which the tutor may have some duty to help. They do not involve supplying an instrument for a crime or anything essential for its commission.

It is arguable that the doctor's conduct is very similar. He provides the contraceptive pills after urging a different course of action, out of a sense of a duty to help. The pills are not an instrument for the crime of unlawful sexual intercourse, nor are they essential for its commission. If, despite that, you find the doctor guilty as an accessory, you will have to find the tutor guilty also, and many other people in similar circumstances. It is doubtful if anyone, even Mrs Gillick, would really wish criminal liability to extend so far.

Woolf J.'s decision in Gillick

Let me now turn to Woolf J.'s judgement in Gillick.[21] Woolf J. made it clear that there *were* circumstances in which a doctor could be guilty as an accessory, if he encouraged the girl or the couple, but regarded such occasions as likely to be very rare. 'I accept', he stated, 'that a doctor who is misguided enough to provide a girl who is under the age of 16, or a man, with advice and assistance with regard to contraceptive measures with the intention thereby of encouraging them to have sexual intercourse is an accessory . . . However, this, I assume, will not usually be the attitude of the doctor.'[22] He agreed with counsel for the DHSS, however, that he could grant the declaration sought by Mrs Gillick only if compliance with the Health Service Notice would *always* constitute a crime. In his judgement, by contrast, the doctor would not commit a crime if he complied with the terms of the Notice and prescribed contraceptive pills only in exceptional cases.

Woolf J. offered three reasons for his judgement. The first is the one that I set out, in different form, above. Woolf J. decided that the contraceptive pills do not directly assist in the crime of unlawful sexual intercourse. 'The analogy of providing the motor car for a burglary or providing poison to the murderer . . . are not true comparisons.' He admitted that the provision of the pills could 'increase the likelihood of a crime being committed', but this, he decided, did not constitute aiding, nor did it amount to encouraging, since encouraging has a subjective, rather than objective, meaning (requiring as it does the appropriate intention). Woolf J. concluded on this point that the prescription of the pill was 'not so much "the instrument for the crime or anything

essential to its commission" but a palliative against the consequences of the crime'.[23]

The second reason offered by Woolf J. was that the girl
commits no crime, so that for the doctor to be guilty as an
accessory, he would have to act through her, as an innocent
agent. This is not, on the present state of legal authorities, an
insurmountable difficulty. Woolf J. was concerned first with the
case in which the doctor saw the girl alone and it was alleged that
he encouraged her to engage in unlawful sexual intercourse. Since
she is the victim of the crime, Woolf J. seems to have taken the
view that it must be the male partner who is encouraged in order
for there to be a crime. Even if this is so, there are cases, for
example *R.* v. *Cogan and Leak*,[24] where it was held that counselling
an *actus reus*, through an innocent agent, can suffice for liability as
an accessory. Alternatively, if it were alleged that the doctor
aided the commission of the crime, the same authorities suggest
that a person may be guilty as an accessory by assisting in the
commission of the crime through an innocent agent. Causing a
child to deliver a jemmy to a burglar friend is an obvious
example. If, then, the doctor could otherwise be guilty as an
accessory, either by encouraging or aiding, the innocent agency
argument would, with respect, probably not save him.

The third ground for Woolf J.'s decision is as follows.

There will be situations where long-term contraceptive measures are
taken to protect girls who, sadly, will strike up promiscuous relationships
whatever the supervision of those who are responsible for their well-
being . . . In such a situation the doctor will prescribe the measures to be
taken purely as a safeguard against the risk that at some time in the
future the girl will form a casual relationship with a man when sexual
intercourse will take place. In order to be an accessory, you normally
have to know the material circumstances. In such a situation the doctor
would know no more than that there was a risk of sexual intercourse
taking place at an unidentified place with an unidentified man on an
unidentified date, *hardly the state of knowledge which is normally associated with
an accessory before the fact*[25] (my emphasis).

The difficulty with this part of the decision is that it does not
seem to accord with the view of the law taken by previous
authorities, nor with the view set out by Woolf J. himself three
months previously, in his judgement in *Attorney General* v. *Able*.[26]

Smith and Hogan summarize the law, which is admittedly complex, as follows, relying on the case of *R. v. Bainbridge*.[27] 'It seems clear that if he [the alleged accessory] knows the type of crime which is contemplated, that would be enough, even if he did not know the person or thing which was to be the subject of it or time, place or other circumstances in which the crime was to be carried out.'[28] In *Able*'s case, Woolf J. had to consider whether supplying a booklet entitled 'A Guide to Self-Deliverance' could constitute a crime, as aiding, abetting, counselling, or procuring the suicide of another, contrary to section 2(1) of the Suicide Act, 1961. Turning to the question of knowledge of the material circumstances, Woolf J. stated 'They would not know precisely when, where or by what means the suicide was to be effected, if it took place, *but this does not mean that they cannot be shown to be accessories*'[29] (my emphasis). All that was needed was knowledge of the type of crime, Woolf J. concluded, citing *R. v. Bainbridge*.[30]

Thus, two of the three grounds on which Woolf J. bases his decision seem, with respect, to be less than convincing. The first ground, the interpretation of the word 'aid', provides the only really sound basis for his judgement that a declaration, in the form required by Mrs Gillick, should not be granted.

To some this may seem a rather unsatisfactory conclusion. For those who support the decision it may seem a fragile basis for the doctor's planning of his future conduct, depending as it does on the flexibilities of one word. The opponents of the decision will also feel dissatisfied, being thwarted, in their eyes, by one word, when everyone knows that words can be put to a number of different uses. In the concluding part of this analysis, I will therefore offer a way out of the legal problem of the possible criminal liability of the doctor, which does not rely on this approach.

An alternative legal analysis

I will state my conclusion at the outset. A doctor is never committing an offence when he is acting as a reasonable doctor. What the reasonable doctor should do, in the sphere of medical ethics, is for all of us to discuss and have our say in determining. Ultimately, it should be set out as the product of a thoughtful and appropriately representative procedure. An example of such a procedure, or at least something that approximates to it, is the publication of the Health Service Notice and accompanying memorandum. It is part of the democratic process, in that it can be challenged and responsible ministers can be called to account for it. It will have been drafted only after consultation with the range of groups and individuals concerned with such matters. Of course, it is not ideal, in that civil servants within any ministry tend to be secretive about whose advice they seek and tend to take power to themselves, and thus become unrepresentative and unresponsive, to the extent that this is allowed (a phenomenon that will be familiar to devotees of 'Yes Minister'). That said, I would suggest that the publication of Codes of Practice or Guidelines is a practice much to be encouraged. In a perfect world, these would be produced by a body adequately representative of the moral and social views of the community. In the interim, a departmental circular open to public scrutiny and challenge is a workable alternative.

Once such a Health Service Notice or Code of Practice or Memorandum is published, those to whom it is addressed, in our case doctors, are entitled to observe it. To do so, the argument goes, would be to act as a reasonable doctor. The Notice would be conclusive on what it is socially and morally permissible for the doctor to do. Those who wish to change the Notice must use the political process and the market-place of ideas. Unless it contained references to law that were contentious, change should not be available through the legal process, provided the proper procedures leading to the formulation of the Notice can be shown to have been observed. For the courts to be granted the power to effect change would, within our constitutional system, be an unwarranted departure from their traditional role as, at best, interstitial legislators unwilling to interfere with or challenge the exercise of properly constituted democratic power. Mrs Gillick would, in other words, have to go to the newspapers and the politicians to change the Health Service Notice and would not be able to go to the courts. The issue would be simply non-justiciable.

The legal way of stating the conclusion just offered is to say that the doctor commits no crime because he has a lawful excuse, derived from his duty to treat. But, of course, the doctor is allowed to deliver only that treatment which is authorized by law. So the argument is in danger of becoming circular. The doctor may treat. But he may treat only if entitled to treat. There is still a need to break out of this circularity and decide whether the doctor's conduct is legally permissible or renders him an accessory.[31]

The way out is to recognize that the doctor's prescription of the pill does fall within the concept of treatment, assuming that there is no intentional encouragement of sexual intercourse. I have suggested already that, as regards the social and moral aspects of treatment, as opposed to the medical-technical, it is for society to mark out the bounds of legitimate treatment. The basis on which the prescription of contraceptive pills may be justified is as follows. Good public policy requires doctors to treat patients for perceived and well-recognized health needs. We are not talking here of any old request from a young girl. What we are considering is a request for contraceptive pills from a girl capable of acting autonomously. One recognized health need relates to the consequences to a girl's health of unprotected sexual intercourse. This health need, and health risk, is an acknowledged fact of life. The doctor, then, is under a duty to treat the girl for this health need by, *inter alia*, prescribing contraceptive pills. It may be that, if he does so, a few girls will be led to engage in sexual intercourse, or to do so more often, when otherwise they would not. But this is simply the inevitable price to be paid for the much greater benefit of maintaining the health of young girls, through a reduction (or at least no increase) in the number of abortions and unwanted pregnancies, and a corresponding reduction in the accompanying ill-health and social cost.

This analysis allows us to solve a problem I posed at the outset, about whether the doctor was entitled to refuse to prescribe the pills or impose unacceptable conditions. If it is accepted that the doctor has a duty to treat, he should be slow to refuse to do so. The duty is one imposed and approved by society. If there is a genuine health risk to the girl, the duty to treat must apply here also. This would mean that the doctor who turned the girl away could well be guilty of neglecting her, should untoward consequences ensue.

Granted, then, that the doctor has this legal duty and assuming that treatment is understood in the way I have suggested, it will follow that he will not be guilty of any crime. He will be behaving as a reasonable doctor, and this for two reasons. First, the reasonable doctor will be the doctor whose sole concern is for the legitimate health needs of, and risks to, his patient. Second, the Health Service Notice and memorandum set out what a reasonable doctor should do, and they accord with what I have suggested concerning the doctor's duty to avoid health risks. The doctor who follows the Notice, therefore, would not be guilty of a crime.

Some authority for the approach I have advocated can be found in Woolf J.'s judgement, even though he does not himself adopt it. He speaks of the case in which the doctor may prescribe contraceptive pills to a girl under sixteen as those in which, 'despite the fact he was firmly against unlawful sexual intercourse taking place . . . [the doctor] felt nevertheless *that he had to prescribe the contraceptives* [as being] *in the best interests of the girl* in protecting her from an unwanted pregnancy and the risk of a sexually transmitted disease'[32] (my emphasis).

Williams also lends authority to my approach when he argues that 'if a person acts in pursuance of a legal duty, (or what would be one but for the law of complicity) . . . he should not be accounted an accomplice'.[33]

The conclusion I arrive at is the same as that reached by Woolf J. The method chosen is, however, very different and in my view to be preferred. It allows for a legal analysis of the doctor's conduct based on the central legal and ethical concept of duty, rather than on the meaning of the 'four traditional verbs'.[34] It allows one to conclude that the doctor should, in matters of moral and social conduct, be guided by documents emanating from properly accountable bodies, and that if he does so he will, quite properly, be insulated from legal liability.

Postscript (February 1985)

I said earlier that it would be nice if the law coincided with what I have proposed as good medical ethics. I then took comfort from the fact (as it seemed to me) that it does. The confidence with which I was then able to state the law has, however, received a cruel blow. Mrs Gillick appealed against Woolf J.'s decision.

After a hearing of five days the Court of Appeal unanimously allowed her appeal (on 20 December 1984). Woolf J. was wrong, the Court decided. The law relating to consent and the rights of parents was not as he stated it.

Not surprisingly, there was much commotion. The Press and television were full of stories praising the decision as reasserting important moral principles, or heralding the doom of unwanted pregnancies and venereal disease which would follow. Many doctors, particularly those involved in family-planning medicine, were dumbstruck and anxiously sought advice on the precise import of the Court's decision.

The dust has not yet settled. Nor will it for a while. The Department of Health and Social Security has decided to appeal to the House of Lords for a final and definitive statement of law.

Without attempting to predict what the House of Lords will decide (and this is one occasion when it would be wiser to hold back with the angels!), it may be helpful to examine analytically the Court of Appeal's judgement. (By the Court of Appeal's judgement, I mean the judgement of Parker LJ, which was the leading judgement.)

Clearly, this is not the place for a detailed exegesis. All I shall attempt is the briefest postscript. It is important, however, to look critically at the reasons offered by the Court for disagreeing with Woolf J. and for reaching a decision which few, if any, commentators thought open to them.

The decision

Put baldly, the Court of Appeal opted for an approach to the issue of prescribing contraceptives to young girls which was couched in the language of parental rights. Parents have rights as regards their children; rights which last at least until a child reaches the age of sixteen. Others may not meddle with these rights. Except in an emergency, only a court can come between parent and child. In particular, a parent has a right to be told of any request a child may make for treatment by a doctor, so as to be able to give or withhold consent. Without such authorization, the doctor is a mere intermeddler, interfering with the legitimate rights of parents, albeit for the best of motives. If he believes that a girl needs care, and that the parents are unjustifiably standing in the way, or would do so if asked, his only recourse is to petition the court. The court can then enquire into the welfare of the child and make whatever decision seems best, which may mean overriding the parents' wishes. The girl cannot give valid consent on her own behalf. The doctor who treats her, without her parents' consent, is therefore not only violating her parents' rights; he is actually assaulting her.

There is obviously a lot to chew on here. What I shall do is divide the argument into its separate components. In so doing, I shall ignore various points concerning administrative and public law, which need not detain us.

Ethical analysis

The Court of Appeal was, of course, at pains to make it clear that its concern was exclusively with the law, and not with moral or social questions. It could not, however, totally avoid taking a view, implicitly or, at times, explicitly, on the rights and wrongs of the issue. For when the law is open (just about) to differing interpretations, the one you choose is the one which best accords with your sense of what is morally right. The Court was clearly persuaded that the interests of family stability, and of the wishes of parents in particular, should prevail over any arguments about a girl's autonomy. That the parents may be perverse or, as evidenced by the child's refusal to involve them, alienated from their child, is no reason for denying them their legitimate moral claims as the child's parents. The Court's model of the parent–child relationship, the child, until the age of sixteen, remaining at home, firmly under the parents' influence and control, clearly bears little relation to the realities of modern life in many households. But the Court, if it was aware of this fact, was quite undeterred by it. Their position appears to have been this: where there is a conflict between what *ought* to be the case and what, as a matter of fact, *is* the case, then it is the facts that must be changed. Reality must be brought into line with what is right. The point that children might have rights too was scarcely even raised, much less conceded. Parents (such was the Court's view) are normally the best arbiters of the interests both of their family and of their children.

This, then, was the ethical base from which the Court

proceeded to state the law. It is an approach which is enjoying a certain vogue at present, representing as it does a reaction against what some see as an over-permissive liberalism.

The capacity of the girl

The legal test of capacity propounded earlier and reflected in Woolf J.'s judgement, was rejected by the Court. They decided that a child under sixteen (and possibly until she reaches majority at eighteen) is under the control of her parents. Consequently, she cannot validly consent to medical treatment, nor can a doctor treat her without parental authority, since otherwise parental rights (on which more later) are violated.

Why, you may ask, did the Court take sixteen to be the crucial age? Well, as regards medical treatment, the Family Law Reform Act, 1969, section 8(1) provides that someone over sixteen may give valid consent. (One has the strong impression that, had that not been the case, parental control would have been said by the Court to last until eighteen.) If the girl over sixteen can consent, then, the Court decided, the girl under sixteen cannot. They purported to derive this from section 8(3) of the same Act, which provides that 'Nothing in this section shall be construed as making ineffective any consent which would have been effective if this section had not been enacted.' This somewhat Delphic utterance had always been assumed to preserve the power at common law of the person under sixteen to give valid consent. The Court, however, tended to the opposite view, that it preserved the common-law power of parents to consent on behalf of their children, even if the child were over sixteen, and to consent on a child's behalf, if she were under sixteen.

The enquiry then turns to what was the common-law position, apart from statute. As I have suggested, virtually every commentator, including me, had no doubt that at common law a person had the capacity to consent, if able to understand what was being consented to. The Court decided otherwise. The common-law rule, they said, was that a child could not give valid consent until she had reached the 'age of discretion', which in the case of a girl was sixteen. In the case of a boy, they said, it was fourteen, apparently unembarrassed by the discriminatory nature of such a rule and the swipe it takes at section 29 of the Sex

Discrimination Act, 1975, which forbids discrimination between sexes in the provision of, *inter alia*, goods and services (including, one might argue, family-planning services).

A number of observations are in order.

1. An analysis of the judgement suggests that it might have either of two implications.

(a) Contraceptive treatment involves contact and conversation between doctor and girl of such a nature that it calls for special rules different from all the normal rules governing medical treatment and other forms of touching consented to by a girl. Its nature is such that a girl under sixteen is intrinsically incapable of validly consenting to it, whatever her capacities in other matters.

This proposition has only to be stated to be shown to be completely untenable, both in fact and in law. There is nothing in the nature of contraception which makes it different in principle from, for example, vaccination, or treatment for vaginal infections or for varicose veins, save for the fact that reproductive functions are involved. But so they are in hormone therapy or the treatment of dysmenorrhea. The judgement cannot, therefore, sensibly be interpreted as making a special case of contraceptive treatment.

(b) Alternatively, the effect goes much further. I have suggested that there is no difference in principle between contraceptive treatment and other medical treatment. Nor can there be between medical treatment and other circumstances in which a girl might be touched with her apparent consent, as in the cases of a handshake, a kiss or embrace, or in a game of netball. If this is right, and it must be in principle, and assuming that the premiss is accepted, then if a girl under sixteen cannot in law consent to contraceptive treatment, it must follow that she cannot in law give valid consent to *any* touching. The kiss and cuddle, the handshake, and so on would equally be unlawful, as being contrary to parental rights, unless consented to by the parent, despite, or regardless of, the girl's consent in fact.

Such a conclusion is, however, contrary both to law and to common sense. Young girls can and do consent to have shoes fitted on them, to have their hair done, or to have cosmetics applied by a shop assistant in a department store. No one, I submit, is breaking the law if he shakes a fifteen-year-old girl's hand, knowing that she was forbidden to see him. Indeed, the law specifically recognizes a young girl's progressive emergence as a person in her own right, as she gains in maturity and understanding. Thus, a girl can be held to her contract, if the contract was for something necessary, such as education, clothes, food, and, significantly, 'physic', as the old writers call it, that is, medical care. The criminal law holds a child responsible for her actions at ten, and under the law of evidence, a child may give evidence if capable of understanding the oath and its significance. Interestingly, the common law requires the enquiry about capacity to be conducted in open court, the judge making the determination after examination.

To argue, therefore, that in none of these cases is the girl of fifteen able validly to consent because she is, by virtue of age alone, disabled from doing so, is to ignore great areas of the common law which say that a girl's capacity to make her own decisions (and mistakes) depends on her understanding, maturity, and intelligence, *not* her age.

2. The age of discretion has always been a rather shadowy notion. It was rather surprising to see it appear, bursting with vitality, in the Court's judgement. Even more surprising was the central importance given to it, such that the Court appeared to regard it as the crucial or clinching argument. It was the age of discretion, the Court said, that the law recognized as the point at which a girl could consent for herself, and that age was sixteen.

The difficulty with this, which did not seem to trouble the Court, is that, historically, the age of discretion was not sixteen for a girl and fourteen for a boy, but twelve for a girl and fourteen for a boy. Until 1929, after all, twelve was the age at which a girl could consent to marry. The age of sixteen is derived from a particular statute, passed in 1549, making it a crime to take girls out of the possession of their fathers. It was an anti-fortune-hunters' statute. The consent of the girl was no defence under the statute.

But this statute, which remains law in a revised form as section 20 of the Sexual Offences Act, 1956, did not state that a girl could not consent to *anything* until sixteen. Indeed, if she had left her father of her own free will and then went off with a man, the man committed no offence and any marriage they subsequently contracted was valid, provided she was over twelve. That a later statute was passed providing that, in such circumstances, she disinherited herself further proves her capacity to consent. So, leaving aside the lack of any real relationship in law or fact between the abduction or seduction of a girl by a man, and her treatment by a doctor seeking only to protect her from health risks, the statutes and cases provide no basis for the Court's conclusion regarding consent and the age of discretion.

Furthermore, in the quite recent case of *R.* v. *D.*, [1984] 3 WLR 186, Lord Brandon, in the House of Lords, specifically decided that, on a charge of kidnapping a child, the prosecution had to show that the child has not consented to go with the person charged. The capacity of the child so to consent was, Lord Brandon went on, dependent not on age, but on whether the child was of sufficient understanding and intelligence to decide for herself. No fixed age, let alone sixteen, got a look-in, though Lord Brandon agreed that at some point the tender age of the child would entitle the Court to assume a lack of capacity. Parliament has since passed the Child Abduction Act, 1984, whereby it is an offence to take a child under sixteen out of the lawful control of a parent, with no mention of consent. But this only confirms that at common law the position was as stated by Lord Brandon.

3. A further reason for fastening on the age of sixteen was the Court's view that the flexible criterion advanced by Woolf J. (and assumed to be the law by the rest of us) was unworkable. First, a doctor would have to make an enquiry of a girl whom he may not know well and whose assurances may not be truthful. He may not, therefore, be in any position to judge. Parents could lose control of their children, and their children's interests could be harmed, on the assessment of some outsider. There would be no certainty in the law, with the result that parents, doctors, and society at large would not know where they stood.

The most obvious response, I suppose, is to point out that doctors have, every day, to assess the capacity of people of whatever age to make decisions, and are trusted to do so. Whether a person is mentally ill, confused, affected by pain, or grief, or drugs, or is simply uncomprehending, is something doctors are already expected and obliged to assess. So the young girl poses no special problem to those trained in family planning and general practice. (Compare, if you will, the assumption that the judge *is* quite competent when it comes to assessing a young person's capacity to take the oath!) Furthermore, a flexible criterion of capacity works in other areas of the law and in other legal systems, such as the Scottish system, which embraces it with no obvious harmful side-effects. In short, it has worked as a criterion in the past and could presumably continue to work. It cannot, therefore, be its lack of apparent certainty that made it objectionable in the eyes of the Court. It must, rather, have been the Court's desire to assert its view of parental rights.

Parental rights

The view of the Court was that a parent has the right to control a girl, even to control her *completely*, at least until she reaches sixteen, and perhaps until the age of majority. This, the Court decided, flows from the right to custody which all parents have over their children. No one may interfere with this right except in emergencies or by order of a court. It follows that a doctor may not treat a girl under sixteen without parental consent, because to do so violates parental rights. A girl may not on her own give a valid consent, as she lacks the requisite legal capacity. The parental right to control entails a lack of capacity in the child, presumably because of some assumed incapacity to know her own best interests until the clock strikes midnight on the eve of her sixteenth birthday.

The Court's decision is, I submit, dubious both as a description of the law and as a description of many (if not most) parent–child relationships, for the following reasons.

1. The basic objection to a decision based on parental rights is that it has always been assumed (and correctly so) that parents have duties towards their children. Whatever rights they have are instrumental only, allowing for the fulfilment of these duties, the primary one being that of bringing a child to maturity and autonomy, free from avoidable harm. If the assertion of a right to control a child's behaviour, in this case her access to a doctor without parental consent, could result in harm to the girl, due to her refusal to involve her parents and the doctor's consequent refusal to treat her, this seems completely at odds with the purpose for which a parent has rights in the first place. Yet this is

the necessary consequence of the Court's decision. To those who argue that the Court's decision strikes a blow not for parental rights but for family stability, by requiring the girl to involve her parents if she wants the doctor to see her, the only answer is to ask them to step back into the real world. Anyone who thinks that family stability can be re-established by *forcing* a girl to talk to her parents, as a condition for receiving treatment, when her conduct in resisting attempts by the doctor to involve them has already shown that family communications are badly damaged, is living in cloud-cuckoo land.

2. The Court placed particular emphasis on the right physically to control a child. In doing so, they chose to be guided by a couple of nineteenth-century cases, and to ignore the changes in law and social attitudes since then, marked both in case law and statute. Lord Denning put it well in *Hewer* v. *Bryant*, [1970] 1 QB 357, when he described the right to control as 'a dwindling right . . . It starts with a right and ends with little more than advice.'

Ever since the nineteenth century, and particularly since 1925, when the Guardianship of Infants Act was passed, statute law has always been concerned to protect not parents' rights, but the best interests and welfare of the child. Furthermore, it is beyond doubt that the idea of a legal right to control must be understood against a background of reality. The law never likes to make itself look silly, by saying you have a right to do what you plainly cannot do, for example chastise your son who happens to be a junior boxing champion. The legal right to control must, therefore, be understood as only enjoyed subject to the extent to which it can be exercised in fact. Thus, as a girl grows up and away from her parents, or the parents lose interest in or neglect the girl (which is often the case as regards contraception), so the legal right to control is lost. It is lost because the duty to bring the child to maturity has either already been fulfilled or else has effectively been abandoned.

3. This brings us to a central objection to the decision. The Court decided that the parent's right to control meant that another, for example a doctor, could not interfere with that right except by first approaching a court, which would then determine the girl's best interests. If parental duties are properly analysed, however, it can be seen that it is the parent who must seek the aid

of the court in matters of control of the child. The parent does not have some presumptive right over a child until sixteen, such that all others must keep their distance. Instead, the parent has the duty to care for the girl, and if he feels that he cannot carry it out because, for example, the girl is turning to someone else, the parent can ultimately ask the court for help. But, significantly, a court will not necessarily side with the parent. It is bound by statute, the Guardianship of Minors Act, 1971, to make the welfare of the child the paramount consideration.

4. A further objection to the Court of Appeal's analysis is that it overlooks the fact that others besides parents may owe duties to the girl. The teacher is one example. His responsibility to the girl may involve doing that which the parent expressly disapproves of, ranging from teaching a subject in a particular way, to encouraging her to enter for an examination, to detaining her for bad behaviour. The doctor equally has responsibilities to a girl who is otherwise capable of consenting to treatment. To give the parental right to control precedence over the various responsibilities of others, particularly when the parent may not properly be exercising that right, is to neglect the welfare of the girl and so violate the policy which has guided family law for more than half a century. To reply that the doctor can always apply to a court, if he feels that the girl is in need of care, is to propose a solution which in practice is no solution at all. Doctors have no time for this, far less the knowledge or appetite. Girls told that they must wait and then go to court will vote with their feet, and the back-street abortionists will rub their hands.

5. It is the final objection, in this brief appraisal, that is perhaps the most telling. The Court of Appeal introduces into the law the notion of a child as a chattel, an object of possession and control. This is hardly the posture that a court, a legal system, or a society committed to the welfare of children would ordinarily adopt. That it contemplates that a parent may refuse consent to treatment which a young girl wants, and a doctor thinks appropriate, is frankly alarming.

The doctor's duty to treat

The idea that a doctor might have a duty to treat, quite apart from parental views, was not raised before the Court. It was, however, implicitly rejected, in that the Court found that a girl had no capacity to give a valid consent until sixteen. Since the doctor needs consent, it therefore follows that he must ask the parent, save in an emergency. Some would like to see this word 'emergency' interpreted very widely, so widely in fact that it would give back to doctors the discretion that the Court has otherwise denied them. It could be argued quite plausibly that every time a girl consults her doctor about contraceptive treatment, it is something of an emergency, since the risk of sexual intercourse and possible pregnancy are very real. Certainly, what I have suggested as good medical ethics could justify giving 'emergency' the widest possible meaning, going far beyond the obvious case of the 'morning after' pill, after unprotected intercourse.

Aside from this, however, the Court appears to give no support to the notion of a duty to treat.

The criminal law

Arguments about possible criminal liability, which were canvassed so vigorously in the High Court, were not greatly pressed or relied upon before the Court of Appeal. What did strike the Court as important was what they took to be the policy reflected in the criminal law's prohibition against sexual intercourse with girls under sixteen. The various crimes were, the Court said, clearly intended to protect a girl from harm and were a clear indication by Parliament that girls were to be protected even from themselves, since although they might consent to sexual intercourse, this consent was no defence for the man. How could it be, the Court asked, that a girl under sixteen was deemed by Parliament to be incapable in law of consenting to sexual intercourse, and yet could consent to contraceptive treatment? The criminal law statutes do exist to protect girls. But the prescription of contraceptives can be seen as entirely in keeping with this Parliamentary policy of protecting them from harm. If sexual intercourse has already taken place or is inevitable, the provision of contraceptives is the only way to protect her from any consequent danger or health risk. To say that she should desist from sexual intercourse may show commendable consistency and commitment, but it ignores the well-recognized fact that sexual intercourse will still take place, contraception or no.

Conclusion

All I have offered are a few brief comments on the Court of Appeal's decision. There are many other things that could be said, but I have chosen to concentrate on an analysis of the issues of principle. Clearly, there is a host of arguments that could be advanced concerning consequences, social, medical, political, and so on. Such arguments might serve to focus attention on the practical implications of our analysis; but they cannot compel any conclusion, although they might help to tip the scales if the analysis and arguments were otherwise finely balanced.

The Court has clearly adopted an ethical stance different from the one I proposed, and has moulded the law accordingly. For the reasons I have indicated, I find the result unsatisfactory on analytical grounds. The case now goes to the House of Lords. Their Lordships have to choose. Clearly, much hinges on their choice; not merely contraceptive treatment and advice, but the whole question of the legal and ethical status of the relationship between parents, children, and others. By the time you read this, the choice will have been made. The House of Lords will have handed down its decision. I, meanwhile, must wait, firmly convinced that the Court of Appeal's view is wrong and that it deserves to be rejected.

3 LITTLE HUMAN GUINEA-PIGS?

R. M. HARE

There is, or at least should be, a close relation between ethical theory and the discussion of practical moral issues. The benefit is mutual. If an understanding of ethical theory (that is, of how to tell good from bad arguments about moral questions) is lacking, our arguments will be reduced to the bandying of one unsupported opinion against another, and victory will go to the side that can command the biggest *claque*. On the other hand, the ethical theorist who neglects to try out his proposals on moral issues of importance is often left maintaining views which would not remain attractive if submitted to this test.

It is very easy, however, to mistake the nature of the test. Some ethical theorists, of an intuitionist and deontological persuasion, (those who base morality on duties which are grasped a priori by intuition), think that they only have to bring their opponents into conflict, on a practical issue, with some commonly held opinion to put them out of court. They would not use such arguments if they reflected that many moral views that are now abhorrent to us have been in some societies almost universally held: for example that cruelty to animals, or even to blacks, does not matter. The appeal to received opinion in support of ethical theory has to be more subtle and more indirect than this. If, at a certain point in history, we find some opinion widely shared, what does this prove? Not that it is correct, as the example just given shows. It indicates, rather, that the reasoning processes used by people in that society lead naturally to such an opinion. The reasoning processes may be at fault. They may be based on ignorance or neglect of relevant facts, and on muddled thinking or the rationalization of self-interested motives.

But if there has been much public discussion of the questions at issue, conducted in the language (*moral* language) that the parties to the discussion have in common, the fact that they have come to this conclusion shows *something* about the rules of this language, which are the rules of argument employing the concepts of the language. If we make the charitable assumption that people do not get their facts wrong all the time, and sometimes think clearly and disinterestedly about moral questions, it is reasonable to hazard the guess that the conclusions they reach are such as can be justified by argument in accordance with these rules, provided that there are no obvious logical muddles or factual mistakes or special pleadings that we can detect. Thus the fact that, when these faults are excluded or allowed for, we can explain the opinions that many thoughtful people come to, and explain them by the hypothesis that they have been arguing, however implicitly or inarticulately, in accordance with certain rules of argument that they accept, shows us something about the rules that they do accept, and thus about the nature of the concepts they are employing; that is, about ethical theory.

So it is always likely to be helpful to the ethical theorist to join in practical moral discussions; and if in return he can help clarify the discussions and expose bad arguments, that is an added incentive. I have myself taken part in many such discussions, often on committees and working parties on such subjects as abortion and euthanasia of which I have been a member, but also in academic seminars. Some of these committees had been set up by the Church of England's Board for Social Responsibility, others under the auspices of the Society for the Study of Medical Ethics. Recently, under the latter's aegis, I took part in a working party on the ethics of research on children, which, like the others, had as its members some distinguished medical people, as well as lawyers, theologians, and philosophers.[1] In the course of preparation for this work, I prepared the list of arguments used for and against particular experiments that is the basis of this lecture. I present it to you as an example of how ethical theory can help moral discussion and vice versa.

It is indeed extremely useful, when faced with a general moral problem of this kind, to draw up such a list. If we put down all the arguments on both sides that we can think of or hear of from others, we have at least some assurance that we have not left out anything that could bear on the question. I drew up the list for the working party, and added to it as new arguments were produced. I then asked myself, in the case of each argument in turn, what sort of argument it was. Was it, for example, an appeal to rights: or was it an appeal to utility? Or was it both—that is to say, was it an appeal to rights, the preservation of which could itself be justified by the utility of preserving them? When all the arguments which seemed in the least acceptable had been sieved out, were there any left that could not be validated in terms of such a utilitarian theory of rights? You will, I hope, see how enormously helpful such an exercise can be in sorting out the dispute between the utilitarians and their opponents. And it helps even more if it is done before a court of practical people who produce real cases in all their specificity, and not before an audience of philosophers who think they can prove points by trotting out fantastic examples with many important details left out.

Before I start on my list of arguments, I must make it clear that I know of no evidence that any clearly objectionable experiments are being done in this country. There was a disturbing case in America some time ago in which children had been deliberately infected in an experiment; but that is not the sort of thing I shall be mainly talking about. There are procedures being used in this country (for example, the taking of blood samples by finger-pricking from children, not for diagnostic purposes) to which, I suppose, nobody would at first sight object, but which *might* be thought to infringe the rights of the child and might also, in extremely rare cases, put the child at some small risk. It is difficult, obviously, to draw a sharp line between this and hypothetical cases in which the risk would not be so negligible, such as a renal biopsy in the course of an operation for some other purpose (where the child, perhaps while having its appendix removed, has a tiny piece of one kidney removed as well, for use in kidney research unrelated to the child's condition). I can well understand the medical profession's desire to have some guide-lines in this area.

So let us start by listing some arguments which might be used *for* a particular piece of research of this kind, or for research on child subjects in general. We have to distinguish between (1) research that is incidental to, and helpful for, the treatment of the particular condition from which the child is suffering (an obvious example being the trying out on the child of a treatment which is still not proved to be a cure for the child's condition, but which may cure him; this is done all the time to both children and adults, and often to their advantage), and (2) research which is not intended in any way to help the patient recover from his condition. An example of this would be the renal biopsy in the case I have just mentioned, where the child had nothing wrong with its kidneys.

The first of these two kinds of research is often called *therapeutic research* and the second *non-therapeutic research*. Some people have thought the distinction between these so important that they have made it the basis of proposed restrictions, saying that non-therapeutic research on children should be banned absolutely. The distinction is not entirely clear, however. Therapy as such—I mean the cure of the individual patient—is never the purpose of research. The two aims are distinct though often combined. If, therefore, we ask for reasons for engaging in research of any kind, the cure of the individual patient cannot be given as one of them. We may hope to learn more about the disease and thus become able to cure *other* patients; but the results of the research, except in extremely rare cases, will not be known until it is too late to use them to help *this* patient.

The key to understanding the distinction between therapeutic and non-therapeutic research is to notice that both research and therapy are marked out as such by their aims, which are different from each other. Research aims at the advancement of knowledge, therapy at the cure of a patient. Therapeutic research cannot be research which is therapy or therapy which is research (that is impossible); it is, rather, an activity which has *both* aims. In the purest case, the very same intervention on a patient may be intended both to cure and to discover something. In less pure cases interventions may take place which have a therapeutic intention but which are modified in some way as an aid to research (for example a few extra millilitres of blood are taken when doing a diagnostic sample, so that the additional blood can be used for research). Therapeutic research is thus an activity which has both aims; non-therapeutic research is an activity which has only a research and not a therapeutic aim.

Why do we carry out research on children, as contrasted with therapy? It is done on humans in general when tests on animals are insufficient to give us the information we need, usually because animals have different physiologies from humans. I must mention in passing that there is of course a very big question about the justification for using animals in experiments; I am not taking up a position on that in this lecture, and shall put the question on one side for the present. Granted, however, that it is all right to use human adults, with their consent, in certain experiments, why use children?

One reason for experimenting on human beings is to test new types of treatment. Now there are some treatments that are applicable only to children, usually because the conditions that they are treatments for only afflict children. Or it may be that a treatment which is suitable and safe for adults is not for children. An example would be if, as is normal, the safe maximum dose for an adult of a certain drug would not be safe for a young child. Or it might be that a much smaller dose was effective for a child; for instance, because the child himself is smaller and therefore the blood-concentration produced by a given dose is larger.

If, therefore, we are to test either the effectiveness or the safety of drugs to be given to children, we may have to try them out on children. Now, as you will know, there are more and less rigorous ways of trying out new treatments. All those with any claim to rigour use control groups; a drug, for example is given to one group and not given to another, and the results compared statistically. In the most rigorous procedure, neither the patients nor those observing the effects of the drug know which patients have had it. In a less rigorous procedure the researchers know but the patients do not. In a still less rigorous procedure everybody knows. The reason for withholding knowledge is to guard against the danger that patients or their doctors may think, or persuade themselves, that they are being helped by a treatment when they are not, or may even be being helped, but only by the so-called 'placebo effect': they think the treatment will help them so they get better, even if the treatment is only doses of coloured water—as happens frequently enough to vitiate tests of drugs if the more rigorous precautions are not observed.

As we shall see, the necessity, in rigorous testing, for these blind and double-blind trials, and the necessity for controls at all, provides one argument *against* experimentation on humans. If some are given just coloured water and no drug, this is depriving them of something which might have helped them. This argument is less strong when one drug is being compared with another (usually a new with an established one); but even here objections can be raised. I should like to mention one example, on the other side, of a case where the omission of controlled tests led to immense harm. At one time paediatricians used to administer oxygen quite freely to new-born babies for various disorders; it helped the disorders and was assumed to be harmless. Only after many years was it discovered that oxygen given in these quantities to neonates can result in their developing a disease of the eyes called retrolental fibroplasia, which is a cause of blindness. If controlled tests had been used from the beginning, the side-effect of the treatment would have been discovered much earlier and a lot of children would not have lost their sight. When it was first suspected that this harmful side-effect was occurring, a controlled trial was done; and this in itself presents ethical problems, because it involved giving the oxygen to some children even though it endangered their sight.[2] I suspect that the same findings could have been achieved statistically by examining past records. A controlled trial at the beginning would not have raised this problem, because then nobody knew, nor was there even any reason to suspect, that oxygen was harmful, and also because, by carefully monitoring its effects, the trial could have been terminated as soon as any adverse ones became apparent. Thus at no time would the researchers have been administering a treatment which they knew, or even had reason to suspect, was other than wholly beneficial. However, this question of the ethics of controlled trials is a subject for a paper by itself, and I shall not pursue it here. Michael Lockwood has written an interesting and provocative paper on the issue.[3]

The other main use of research on children (as on adults) is entirely non-therapeutic; it is where in order to study certain abnormalities properly (for example, deficiency diseases like rickets) we have to know what is the normal value of a certain variable—what, say, is the normal amount of a certain substance in the blood of children in a given population. Only then can we know what variations are departures from the normal, and which are significant. One could not combat rickets in a population of children safely and effectively without this information. More generally, the acquisition of new knowledge in medicine is bound to require the doing of various things to human bodies; and some of these things cannot be done without interventions which, if made without consent and outside the medical context, would count as assaults. Some of these are quite trivial like the taking of blood samples and the testing of knee-jerks; others, like the renal biopsies I mentioned, are more serious. If, however, we think the advance of medical knowledge to be on the whole in the general interest, and agree that it would be to some degree hampered if such interventions were forbidden, this may make us ready to allow them in at least some cases.

So far I have been talking of the reasons that could be given for using children as subjects which arise from the advance of the research itself. Next we must consider some benefits which the children themselves may get out of the research. I am not speaking of benefits to other children who may be cured as a result of the development of the treatment; that has already been covered. But the child himself who is the subject may, as a result, get a new drug which may cure him, when the drug, because it has not yet been fully tested or because it is not yet mass-produced, is not generally available. We have only to think of the great efforts that some cancer patients have made to obtain interferon, even though it was not yet known to be effective against cancer of any sort. There are certainly conditions under which I would allow myself to become a research subject for that reason; and I would also allow my child to be, at least if the child were dying.

Then there are certain quite extraneous reasons why one might wish to become a subject—reasons which a child also might acknowledge, if he were able to understand what was going on. First, suppose that some handsome payment is given for a quite trivial intervention. There are obvious dangers in hiring children as research subjects; it puts temptation in the way of their parents. But I do not think that these dangers should altogether rule out the practice. Other incentives, such as giving badges to children who surrender their baby teeth when they fall out so that the teeth can be used for research, seem relatively harmless. This is perhaps the place to mention what we might call the moral inducement: we might say that we all, including children, have a duty to help our fellow humans, and one way we can do this is by furthering the progress of medical research. So if I allow myself to be used as a research subject, I am adopting one way of fulfilling this duty. If an older child did this voluntarily, knowing what he was doing, then it would be one up to the child; we should think of him as we do of voluntary blood donors. This inducement is not applicable to young children; but it has been suggested (not by me) that it is not unreasonable to expect them to do their duty by the community if there is something which they alone can do, and at very small cost to themselves.

The last category of pro-arguments that I shall consider will raise eyebrows; but I include it for the sake of completeness. Both the researcher and his institution get benefits from the research if successful (and sometimes even if not). His knowledge and skill is improved; so is the reputation of the institution. This may produce financial advantages by advancing the career of the researcher or the attractiveness of the institution to funding bodies. Though there are obvious dangers in these motives, and they have led to research of all sorts being carried out which ought not to have been, the motives are not in themselves bad. They need some measure of control; but in the absence of counter-arguments they would be perfectly respectable.

That, then, is the end of my list of pro-arguments. It may not be complete. But what are the considerations on the other side? First, it can be said that almost any intervention in somebody's body carries a risk, however trivial, of discomfort, danger to health or even to life. This applies even to things like taking blood samples. Using anybody as a research subject therefore needs justification. This is seen most easily in the case of non-therapeutic research, where there is no intended benefit to the subject's condition. It may be that the benefits to society through the advance of research will outweigh the danger, but this needs to be shown.

Even in the case of therapeutic research, where the patient may benefit through possible cure, there are still difficulties. First, if the treatment is new, it may have undesirable and unexpected side-effects. Or it may turn out to be less effective than an older treatment, and in research it is not usually possible to give both at once. If, in a controlled trial, a placebo is used for the control group, then, as we saw earlier, the patients in that group are being denied, through their bad luck in being in that group and not in the group which receives the treatment, the chance of benefiting from it. This unfairness is not so apparent where a new treatment is being compared with an old, as is much more common; but even here there is the likelihood that one treatment will turn out to have been better than the other, so that the ones who got the worse treatment were disadvantaged. On the other side, it could be said that, since it was not known in advance which treatment would turn out better, both groups were given an equal *chance* of benefit. This argument could even be used with placebos in cases where there is no alternative treatment: those who get the treatment get a chance of cure and a chance of harm through side-effects; those who get the placebo get neither, but the risks they avoid and the benefits they lose may exactly balance out. However, this is unlikely always to be the case.

It would seem that all these counter-indications apply at least as much to child subjects as to adults, if not more. There are others which apply especially to children. To take the simpler ones first: children are easily frightened, and it is often difficult or impossible to explain to them what is going on. They may find themselves taken in charge by strange people and subjected to procedures whose effects and whose purpose they know nothing about; they may not know from one moment to the next what is going to happen to them. Children usually make a fuss about injections even when attended by loving parents and handled by the most kindly doctors and nurses; great benefits obviously have to be claimed before it becomes justifiable to subject children to these traumas. The same would apply even more forcefully to any procedure which involved separating children from their parents when it was not necessary for their treatment. For all these reasons it may be wrong to do to a child what it would be perfectly all right to do to an adult with his consent.

But it is this question of consent which makes the biggest difference between adults and children. It is generally held, and is held by the law, that children below certain ages cannot give valid consent for certain things to be done to them. This is on several grounds. First, it is held that consent requires full information about what is being consented to; and this children, if they cannot understand what is to be done to them, do not have. There is obviously a gradation here; a new-born baby knows absolutely nothing, but a fifteen-year-old may have a very good idea—perhaps better, if he is intelligent, than some less intelligent adults.

Secondly, consent requires that the consenter is free to refuse; but this can mean two things at least. In one sense a person is not free if you tie him to the operating table, or administer an anaesthetic without his knowledge, and cut him up. In a different sense he is not free if he is subject to threats of some evil or other if he will not consent. For example, his parent may say he will give him a whipping if he will not. I am going to call this 'duress'. It needs to be asked whether children necessarily lack freedom in any of these ways. I think it can be taken for granted that if a child, or anybody else, is ignorant or physically manhandled, he does not consent freely. Duress is more tricky. The illustration I gave is clear enough. But what if the parent is in the habit of giving the child sweets and says the sweets will stop if the child does not consent? What, on the other hand, if the parent is *not* in the habit of giving the child sweets, but says that he will on this occasion if the child consents? Lawyers can say more about this; but I shall not. If the bride tells the bridegroom that she will not marry him unless he promises that the children of the marriage will be brought up in the Roman Catholic religion, has he consented freely if he so promises? If I am told that I cannot have the car unless I pay £3,000, and consent to pay it, is my consent free?

Though this is a murky area, some things can nevertheless be said about it. It seems safe to say that at any rate some children on whom experiments of minor sorts might be performed cannot consent validly to them. This must be the case with new-born babies. Are we to ban such experiments altogether because valid consent cannot be given? The reasons for the inability to give valid consent are the very same reasons that make us protect children by keeping them—so long as and to the extent that these reasons hold—under the tutelage of their parents or guardians. Because children lack knowledge of the effects of their actions and of what is done to them, we to a greater or lesser extent allow parents to decide for them what they may do or what may be done to them; the parents supply the knowledge which the children lack. Similarly with freedom; because children are weak and therefore at the mercy of force and duress, we keep them under the protection of parents, who can prevent unauthorized persons submitting them to such force or duress, but who are themselves allowed to apply force or duress for what they think is the child's own future good.

For these two reasons—the child's lack of knowledge and of freedom—parents normally make and enforce a great many decisions for their children. The question in the present case is whether these decisions may rightly include decisions to let the child be experimented on. In order to answer this question, we have to ask more generally why there should be a right, even of adults, not to have things done to their bodies without their consent. I fancy that it is here that an apparent division will come to the surface between utilitarians and their intuitionist opponents—a division which I hope to have shown elsewhere to be only apparent.[4]

Some people will claim that there just *is* this right; we all know it exists and no reason needs to be given for it. I do not myself belong to this school of thought, because I like to have reasons for what I say—it comes in so handy when others disagree with one. The grounds on which I would defend this right are utilitarian. It seems generally to be the case that normal adults are better judges of their own future good (their own interest) than other people who may think they know better. It is in this belief that we seek to protect people from interference, however well meant, by other people. This protection we give by acknowledging and preserving a right to non-interference, and entrenching it or hedging it about with very strong moral feelings (what Sir Stuart Hampshire, a notable intuitionist, calls 'outrage or shock'[5]) if ever the right is infringed. So, even if our reasons for according the right are utilitarian, we do want people, ourselves included, to have these intuitions, and normally to act on them without hesitation, rather than sickly them over with the pale cast of thought, which may lead us into all kinds of special pleading (particularly if the experiment is important to our career), and in any case will be based on knowledge which, though it may be greater than the patient's, is a great way from omniscience, and may be quite insufficient for forming a wise opinion. We do better in most cases to stick to our moral convictions, provided that these are in general sound ones.

However, once we see the reason for acknowledging this right, we see also that it is only a right in general, or prima facie; it is, as I think the lawyers say, defeasible. Even if, for practical reasons, we want, as we should want, to keep our moral principles manageably simple, there may be certain broad classes which we make into exceptions to a principle. For example, we all think killing people is wrong, but most of us think that it is all right to kill somebody if that is the only way of stopping him killing us. The question for us here is 'Given that in general we acknowledge a right not to have one's body interfered with without one's consent, ought the right to be relaxed in the case of some children? Ought, therefore, the well entrenched general rule to have an exception of some sort written into it, allowing some kinds of research on children without their own consent? And if so, in what sorts of cases, and under what conditions? In particular, if the children cannot give consent, who should be required to give it?'

Since consent is required from adults because that is thought to be in general the best way of securing their interests, we have to ask what is the best alternative way of securing the interests of children who cannot give consent. An extreme way might be to forbid all experiments on children. An only slightly less extreme way would be, as some have suggested, to forbid all non-therapeutic research on them. But this would be in some cases to forgo great benefits to the advance of medicine in order to avoid negligible harms to subjects. Most of us are utilitarians to this extent, that if, by pricking some children's fingers to take blood samples, we could produce crucial evidence which would lead to the elimination of a disease that killed large numbers of children, we would think it reasonable to allow the children's parents to give consent to the experiment on the children's behalf. Such a widespread opinion in itself proves nothing, except that in such a case the utilitarian verdict is not wholly counter-intuitive.

If it were a case of adults, we might reason as follows: the benefits that come from the experiment are likely to be very great; the discomfort and risk to the subjects are extremely small; so, although the adult should have a *right* to withhold consent, it would be wrong of him to exercise that right. In the case of a child who cannot give or withhold consent, the same considerations apply at one remove. For the same reasons as we give to adults a right to refuse consent (namely because we think that that is the safest thing in the interests of adults generally), we give children a right not to be interfered with without the consent of their parents (because that is the safest thing in the interests of children generally). But for the same reason as we say that it would be wrong for an adult to refuse consent in a case like this (because the benefit hoped for is very large and the risk extremely small), we say that it would be wrong for a parent, whose consent is made a condition in order to protect the interest and the right of the child, to refuse it (because, again, the benefit is large and the risk small). This result could easily be reversed if the benefit were smaller or more unlikely, or the risk greater. The whole question is therefore going to turn on the quantification of these risks and benefits. Our working party's report will have a whole chapter on risks and their quantification.

Since there is obviously going to be some quantification of risks and benefits to be done, it will never be sufficient, even in the case of adult subjects, to leave the decision simply to the researcher and the subject between them. For the researcher is an interested party, and the subject, if a layman, may not have, and may not even be able to understand, the information which is required for a rational decision. The same applies to parents making such decisions on behalf of their children. That is one reason, though not the only one, why hospitals and research institutions ought to have ethical committees containing disinterested experts who can look at the details of proposed experiments and see whether the benefits do exceed the risks by a sufficient margin. Since all experiments are different, general guidelines in writing cannot achieve this, necessary as they are. A parent making such a decision ought to have the safeguard of knowing that such a committee has passed the experiment, even if he cannot himself weigh up the benefits and risks as an expert can.

Another reason for having ethical committees is that they can look at these questions continuously over a period of time, and thus gain experience, and so perhaps be able to lay down for themselves and others general guidelines, so that experiments will not even be proposed which the committees would be unlikely to permit. They can also exercise a general surveillance to see that the rights of children and their parents are not being infringed, or, if they are, to make recommendations which, if such abuses turn out to be widespread, may lead to a tightening of the law.

I have said that such committees should contain experts, as obviously they must if they are to understand what they are deciding. Ought they also to contain laymen with special qualifications? The same question applies to any *national* bodies that advise or adjudicate on such questions. Or ought there to be two kinds of committee, one consisting of experts and the other at least partly of laymen? That was the solution proposed in Florida to look after a similar problem—the regulation of the use of behaviour therapy in prisons and mental hospitals.[6] It has been suggested in this country that there should be, in addition to the General Medical Council, which is an expert body, a different body consisting in part of experts in medicine but in part of practitioners of other relevant disciplines like law, and of others experienced in the problems that arise. Our own working party had, of course, such a composition, and so have many similar *ad hoc* and temporary committees and commissions, some enjoying a more official status than others. The suggestion is that there should be a *permanent* body of this sort for all problems arising in medical ethics and bioethics.[7] Apart from a fear that its proceedings might become too congested if it took on so much, and that it would have to proliferate subcommittees to cope with various specialist fields, I have nothing in principle against the proposal. But I can conceive of some doctors objecting.

Obviously there is a lot more to be said about possible procedures. But the most useful thing our working party did was to discuss questions of principle, illustrating the principles by considering real cases. We were able by this means to display, and even to some extent quantify, the factors that are important in such decisions. This paper has consisted of a list of these factors without any attempt at quantification; but we thought it possible for those engaged in research to give an idea of how important each factor is in a selection of typical cases, and so enable us to devise a set of helpful guidelines. This is what our working party has tried to do.

In conclusion, it will have been noticed that all the pros and cons that I listed were of a broadly utilitarian sort. I tried hard to include every reason, whether utilitarian or not, that anyone could suggest for or against conducting such experiments; but it turned out that all the sustainable reasons were compatible with utilitarianism, even those which had to do with the rights of children and parents.

It is worth while to emphasize this point. Looking at the surviving reasons again, it seems to me that the only ones that are not obviously utilitarian are those concerned with unfairness to control groups who do not get a drug which might have benefited them, and those concerned with a right not to be experimented on without one's consent. I hope I have shown in the latter case that the requirement of consent has a utilitarian justification, as has the allowing of proxy consent, with safeguards, in the case of children. As regards unfairness to control groups, I have not discussed the question fully; but two points can be made. One is that, as I have argued elsewhere, there is an adequate utilitarian justification for our insistence on justice in general and on the particular principles of justice that most of us accept. To put it baldly, things go much better in a society where such principles are respected. The other is that in actual cases of research, as opposed to fictional ones, it should be possible to observe these principles without invalidating the research. Certainly there are nearly always both advantages and disadvantages in belonging to the control group, and so it is not treated unfairly. If the same requirement of consent or proxy consent is imposed in controlled experiments as in others, the subjects in the control group can have their interests protected. For the fact that he is taking part in the experiment will be known either to the subject himself or to the proxy consenter (though neither may know which group the subject has been assigned to). So consent can be refused if being a control seems not to be in the subject's best interests. It would be wrong if such a refusal resulted in the withholding of therapy altogether; but I assume that this is not in question.

So I was left at the end of the working party convinced that a carefully constructed utilitarian system of the sort that I advocate can handle an issue like this in a way that does justice to the intuitions and convictions that most of us have, or at least to those which we shall retain when we have reflected sufficiently on the issue.

4 THE ETHICS OF COMPULSORY REMOVAL

J. A. MUIR GRAY

In recent years there has been considerable debate about the compulsory removal from their homes of people who are mentally ill. The debate has focused on a number of different issues: how mental illness should be defined, who should be responsible for removal, and what safeguards should exist for the protection of the individual. With the exception, however, of a very few radicals such as Thomas Szasz,[1] there is general acceptance of the need for such powers, because it is generally accepted that there is a condition of mind, still most usefully defined by the old-fashioned term 'insanity', which ethically justifies paternalistic interventions such as the compulsory removal of someone from his home. There is, though, another piece of legislation in the United Kingdom which has received much less attention in recent years, although it is ethically far more contentious. This is Section 47 of the National Assistance Act which allows for the removal of individuals who are not insane and for their compulsory detention in institutions.

Section 47 of the 1948 National Assistance Act gave the Medical Officer of Health the power to apply to a magistrate for the compulsory removal of persons who

(a) are suffering from grave chronic disease or, being aged, infirm or physically incapacitated, are living in insanitary conditions, and (b) are unable to devote to themselves, and are not receiving from other persons, proper care and attention.

Section 47 also allows the Medical Officer of Health to use these powers to remove a person to prevent 'injury to the health of, or serious nuisance to, other persons'. To obtain an order for removal the Medical Officer of Health had to give seven days' notice to a Court of Summary Jurisdiction which could authorize a person's 'detention' for a period not exceeding three months in a 'suitable hospital or other place'.

In 1951 this Act was amended to allow for the immediate removal of individuals who could not be left for seven days. The legislation was amended because of the fate of one woman who lay on her kitchen floor for the seven-day period of notice required by the 1948 Act and who during that time developed a pressure sore which became infected with tetanus bacteria, with the result that she died of tetanus. The powers of immediate removal were obviously open to abuse because the legislation allowed for a Justice of the Peace to grant an order in his own home and did not require the Medical Officer of Health to approach a court. To safeguard the rights of the individual the Medical Officer of Health was required to obtain the support of another registered medical practitioner and was allowed to apply for removal only for a period of three weeks' 'detention'.

With the reorganization of the National Health Service in 1974, the responsibility for the execution of these powers passed from the Medical Officer of Health to the community physician. The legal power is still invested in the District Council, which is also responsible for environmental health, but the community physician acts as the 'Proper Officer' to the District Council.

These powers are infrequently used. Only about 200 people are removed annually. In most cases the powers of immediate removal are employed and the great majority of individuals removed are elderly. These 200 cases are, however, only the tip of the iceberg. Many more are referred to community physicians and are not removed; and there are many more old people who are either at risk or who are neglecting themselves who are not referred and who are either left at home at risk or in a state of dirt and disorder, or whose admission is effected by one means or another. The elderly person may, for example, be coerced into accepting hospitalization by the unremitting pressure of her relatives and professional advisers. She may be deceived by being told that she is only 'going for a holiday' when she is in fact being admitted permanently to a home or her resistance may be overcome by tranquillizing drugs. In one case in which Section 47 was not used the general practitioner simply added a powerful tranquillizer to the old person's tea.

Self-neglect

It is common for people to take less care of their appearance as they grow older, for example to buy fewer new clothes or to go to the hairdresser less frequently. For the majority of people this trend simply reflects the fact that income usually declines on retirement and the fact that many people become less vain about their appearance as they grow older.

There is, however, a small proportion of people who seriously neglect themselves and their dwellings. The common pattern is for the individual to wear old clothes and to live in a cluttered and dirty house surrounded by an unkempt garden. The precise pattern differs from individual to individual. (Personally, I tend to divide such cases into those with cats, and those without.) Some maintain personal cleanliness; while others become dirty and begin to smell. Some simply wear old clothes, whereas others wear torn and filthy ones. Some simply preserve newspapers, books, and papers; others have piles of mouldering food and rows of unwashed milk bottles. Some seek medical attention when they become unwell; others fail to do so.

It has been suggested that all individuals who neglect themselves are suffering from the 'Diogenes syndrome';[2] but this term is a reflection more of the desire of the medical profession to classify individuals, than of the objective existence of any such condition. Individuals who neglect themselves and their environment have only this feature in common; they are no more likely to be similar in other respects than are any two individuals selected at random.

Old people at risk

Elderly people who neglect themselves are often at risk: risk of hypothermia, risk of falling, or risk of fire. But there are other individuals who do not neglect themselves in any way other than in failing to take appropriate steps to reduce the risks they run, for example the clean and well-dressed elderly person who lives in a neat and tidy house but who refuses to use more than one electric fire in the winter, even though he has previously been admitted to hospital suffering from hypothermia.

Old people who are deemed to be 'at risk' are the subject of considerable public and professional concern. They, like elderly people who neglect themselves, are frequently referred to consultants in geriatric medicine or psychiatrists or to community physicians. Referrals to the latter are often accompanied by requests for compulsory removal.

Refusal of help

The fact that an elderly person is at risk or neglecting herself does not by itself constitute an ethical problem. There are two things that make it a problem: first, the old person's refusal of offers of help, and secondly the beliefs and attitudes of other people, which determine the ethical context in which the professional has to work and make his decisions.

The beliefs of elderly people help to influence their attitudes towards and decisions about help and treatment. Some elderly people believe that all their problems are caused by the ageing process and are *ipso facto* untreatable. Alternatively, the elderly person may accept that his problem was at one time treatable, but believes that it is now 'too late' or even—a commonly expressed view—that the health and social services should not waste their resources on elderly people: as one old woman who was refusing help put it, 'Help those handicapped children who are in much greater need than I am.'

It is important to appreciate the strength of these beliefs and not simply to see them as a form of ignorance. In many cases the elderly person has a very solid foundation for his or her beliefs:

Miss S. was house-bound and immobilized by Parkinson's disease and arthritis. She was referred to the community physician because she consistently refused to heat her house other than by one storage heater. The community physician visited her on a cold frosty February morning. The window of the room in which the old person was sitting was open and cold fog was drifting into the room. All the community physician's arguments about why the old person should be using more heating were politely received but obviously made no impact. As he was on the point of leaving, the old lady said 'I used to work for your predecessor, the Medical Officer of Health.' When questioned she revealed that she had been a schoolteacher in the school for delicate children forty years previously, working in an era in which the medical profession advocated cold fresh air as a vitally important prophylactic and therapeutic measure.

Yet another reason why many elderly people say 'What else can you expect at my age?' is that at some time or other some doctor has said to them 'What else can you expect at your age?'[3]

Religious beliefs are also important. Some elderly people are fatalistic, believing that their problem has been sent by God or that God has let it happen; that it is a manifestation of God's will. Fortunately this does not usually lead to a refusal of offers of help and treatment, because they too are seen as manifestations of God's will. Of greater importance is the fact that some older people interpret their suffering as a punishment for some past sin, basing their belief on the Prayer for the Sick in the Book of Common Prayer. On occasion, an elderly person becomes pre-occupied with her guilt and for this reason is not interested in offers of help.

In some cases shame at the condition into which she has drifted leads an old person to bar her house to those who would help her:

Miss N. was the only surviving sister of three who had once lived in a large house. She now lived in the basement of the house and had consistently refused offers of help when these were suggested by a neighbour who did all her cooking and shopping. One December evening the neighbour felt unable to continue her support and asked the general practitioner to visit. He found Miss N. sitting on the floor of her basement, her face and hands dirty; she was cold and blue, showed signs of early hypothermia and congestive cardiac failure, and her left foot was lying in an awkward position suggesting a fractured neck of femur. She refused the offer of hospital admission and the community physician had her compulsorily removed from her cold and filthy basement. She sobbed as she was removed, the tears coursing through the dirt that was thick on her cheeks.

An hour after admission, after she had been bathed and changed, she smiled and waved at the community physician and said that the reason she had been unwilling to accept help was that she had become ashamed of the condition into which she had allowed herself to slip.

Self-neglect may of course be a sign of depression, with the elderly person feeling himself worthless and useless and perhaps wishing to die. There are, however, elderly people who want to die who cannot be said to be depressed; for example, elderly disabled people who find their lives intolerable or pointless and who wish to be released. Such people rarely actively refuse offers of treatment, though. Usually they accept passively the help that is given, often expressing the wish that they would die and cease to be a burden on those who help them.

Incompetent old people

If an old person is neglecting herself or allowing herself to be at risk because she is suffering from a severe degree of dementia, or a severe degree of depression, she can be considered to be insane and the Mental Health Act can be used to remove her from her home to a hospital. But what about the very many elderly people who have either a milder degree of dementia or some other disease that causes intellectual impairment, for example alcoholism? These people cannot be removed using the Mental Health Act, for when interviewed they are quite obviously not severely mentally ill and would not, in the opinion of a reasonable person, be considered to be insane; but nor would they be considered by the man on the Clapham omnibus to be completely normal. Individuals such as this may be considered to be incompetent.

The concept of incompetence is, like the concept of insanity, a legal concept. But unlike the latter it does not refer to the individual's mind as a whole but only to the individual's ability to use his mind in certain specific situations. As Beauchamp and Childress put it,

Some persons who are legally incompetent may be competent to conduct most of their personal affairs, and vice versa. The same person's ability to make decisions may vary over time, and the person may at a single time be competent to make certain practical decisions but incompetent to make others. For example, a person judged incompetent to drive an automobile may not be incompetent to decide to participate in medical research, or may be able to handle simple affairs easily, while faltering before complex ones.[4]

I, for example, would not be competent to hold the post of Professor of Mathematical Logic.

Most of the case law on competence is concerned with the validation of wills. For the will to be valid the testator must be of testamentary capacity. The decision that a person is not of testamentary capacity has to be made by a solicitor who has been asked to help the person make his will. The solicitor will, of course, take into account medical information; but the decision that a person is incompetent is a legal decision. Interestingly, the fact that a person has been compulsorily admitted to a psychiatric hospital, and may therefore be considered to be insane, does not necessarily imply that he is also incompetent and therefore unable to make a valid will. It is true that medical advice is of importance, and indeed a study of the definition of incompetency in New York State 'revealed that labelling replaced analysis and that the real decision-maker albeit by default was the examining physician . . . [S]eldom is any attempt made to enquire into the actual manner in which the disease affected economic value judgements.'[5]

Determining incompetence is relevant both in situations in which the individual is deemed to be at risk and in situations in which he is either neglecting himself or refusing the offer of effective treatment. Numerous referrals are made to the health and social services concerning elderly people who are deemed to be at risk of setting fire to their dwellings; and indeed it is true that the mortality rate from fire is higher in old age, increasing from 3 deaths per 100,000 per annum in the age group 65–74 to 15 deaths per 100,000 per annum in people aged over 85. Requests for the compulsory removal of individuals who are refusing admission to hospital for treatment are common, in spite of the fact that Section 47 does not give doctors the power of treatment, but only the power of removal. Even if a person were to be removed using Section 47, the doctor in hospital who treated that person against his will could still be charged with assault. This is less of a problem in practice, however, than it is in theory. I have admitted six people compulsorily to hospital, all of whom have required treatment of one sort or another, and all accepted the treatment without explicit refusal. This was either because they ceased their opposition to hospital treatment once hospital admission had been effected, or because they simply complied with the expectations of firm, polite, and busy hospital staff who were in many cases unaware of the difficulties that preceded admission. Hospital staff do not, after all, ask the patient for his consent every time they have to perform a test or give treatment: compliance is assumed once the person has been admitted to hospital.

The attitudes and beliefs of other people

The attitudes and beliefs of other people influence the behaviour of the old person, the timing and nature of the referral, and the behaviour of the professionals involved. In these attitudes and beliefs, genuine care and concern are typically combined with an underestimation of the ability of elderly people to assess the risks they are running. Hence there is a general assumption that elderly people should be protected from the consequences of their actions.

For example, in the debate on Section 47 of the National Assistance Bill in the House of Commons the Minister of Health stated that it was self-evident that

where an old person is living in a house and is utterly incapable of looking after himself, who has no-one at all who can look after him, and where such people are in a very bad state of health and sanitary condition, some authority must be responsible for looking after them and someone must do something about it. It is in the interests of the old people themselves that this power is taken and not in the interests of a tyrannical state.[6]

The Minister of Health stated that something 'must' be done, and no one disagreed. For there is a general assumption that very elderly people who act atypically are not competent, a belief that probably stems in part from the belief that all very elderly people are suffering from dementia; whereas in fact only a minority of old people develop this disease.

The greatest pressure on the old person and the attending professionals often comes from neighbours and relatives who feel guilty. For the person who feels guilty as a result of the condition in which he sees one of his elders and wants to alleviate his guilt, the choice is simple: either he must provide practical assistance for the old person, or else he must attempt to have the old person removed from his sight to be 'looked after' or 'cared for', thus removing the object of his guilt. Some people still feel morally outraged if a person is neglecting himself, because they feel that this neglect is tantamount to suicide by an act of omission, and as such is as wrong, morally, as suicide by an act of commission. In this context, it is important to remember that when the legislation which became Section 47 (Section 56 of the Bradford Corporation Act of 1925) was first drafted, suicide was a crime, and was still regarded by many people as a grave sin.

Similarly, calls for the removal of elderly people, which were articulated first at the end of the nineteenth century and in the majority and minority reports of the Poor Law Commission in 1909, reflected not only concern about the individual but also a general concern about the effects of dirt and disorder on society as a whole. People's attitudes towards dirt and disorder, and also to incontinence, make a fascinating study in themselves. Clearly, people have traditionally felt threatened by them (though, of course, individuals differ widely in their level of tolerance of dirt and disorder). Societies depend on a degree of order if they are to survive. And dirt is merely one form of physical disorder. Our reactions to the old person who is living in filthy conditions may in part reflect the fear, at some deep level of our psyche, that disorder may engulf us. (Or even a fear that we may willingly succumb to it. From one point of view, order and cleanliness exercise, for most of us, a kind of tyranny; the person who is incontinent and lives in squalor has, in a sense, cast off the yoke. He therefore evokes in us the anxiety that is the conscious manifestation of a repressed desire to do likewise.) Of course there are now known to be sound medical and biological reasons for wishing to avoid some forms of dirt; but the anxiety that dirt has traditionally aroused can hardly be attributable to that, seeing that our forebears knew nothing of the connection between dirt and disease (unless, as some sociobiologists might claim, our aversion to dirt and physical disorder in general could be shown to have an evolutionary explanation). I would suggest, at any rate as an historical matter, that Section 47 has had, as one implicit objective, that of imposing order and cleanliness, not merely as a way of protecting others from some palpable threat, such as that of disease, but for its own sake: because deviance in these respects offends and disturbs us. In short, I believe that there is an element here of using the law in a way that was defended, in opposition to the Wolfenden Report,[7] by Lord Devlin: namely for the enforcement of society's morals.[8] Devlin's thesis provoked some celebrated rebuttals, most notably from Herbert Hart;[9] but I shall not rehearse the arguments here.

At any event, one still encounters strong feelings about elderly people who are living in a state of dirt and disorder. Sympathy for the elderly person is mixed with fear, on the part of the neighbours who are worried about fire, and with the anger of those who feel that the old person could do more to help himself if he tried:

Miss S. had lived all her life in a small village. She was now nearly seventy and lived in a small almshouse, the door of which faced that of a neighbouring almshouse, a mere four feet away. The floors of her dwelling were two feet thick in hard-packed dirt; and for light she relied on paraffin which she kept by her front door in open containers. Her clothes and her person were dirty and in the summer both she and her house stank.

It was decided not to remove her from her house, but to dig out the dirt. In order to facilitate this, her furniture was temporarily removed and stored in the village hall. The result was that the hall keeper and several members of the hall committee resigned in protest; and it became clear that although a number of villagers thought it wrong that help had not been offered this lady earlier, others in the village, while conceding that she was of limited intelligence, felt that it was wrong to use public money to help her at all. This in view of the fact that she was, for example, still able to take the bus to a neighbouring town to play bingo, and indeed occasionally won.

The history of witchcraft is very illuminating in helping us understand the feelings aroused by the elderly poor. The subjects of witchcraft allegations were not, as is sometimes supposed, usually people affected by what we would now call schizophrenic or hysterical states; they were most often poor elderly women, as is pointed out by Keith Thomas in his brilliant book *Religion and the Decline of Magic*.[10] The social context in which accusations were made was one in which social relationships were changing: the manorial system, which 'had done much to cater for widows and elderly persons by a built-in system of poor relief', was in decline, 'population pressure eroded many of the old customary tenancies and led to the taking in of the commons and the rise of competitive rents'.[11] Two other factors were of great significance. The Reformation removed a very effective means, in the confessional, of allaying guilt, while the institution of a national Poor Law, which 'set up overseers of the poor, charged with levying a rate and making provision for the dependent members of the parish, . . . sap[ped] the old tradition of mutual charity . . . Nothing', Keith Thomas observes, 'did more to make the moral duties of the householder more ambiguous.'[12] He concludes:

This uneasy conjunction of public and private charity exacerbated the uncertainty with which contemporaries viewed the poor. They hated them as a burden to the community and a threat to public order. But they also recognised that it was their Christian duty to give them charity when no public relief was forthcoming. The conflict between resentment and a sense of obligation produced the ambivalence which made it possible for men to turn begging women brusquely from the door, and yet suffer torments of conscience after having done so.[13]

The tensions that produced witchcraft allegations were thus those generated by a society which no longer held a clear view as to how its dependent members should be treated; they reflected the ethical conflict between the twin and opposing doctrines that those who did not work should not eat and that it was blessed for the rich to support the poor.[14]

The same situation obtains today. People are uncertain where neighbourly help stops and professional help starts. Members of the public see social problems in their society and maintain that professionals should do the caring but feel guilty that they themselves are not caring, just as in seventeenth-century England —with one difference. The accusations are no longer directed at the poor elderly people themselves but at the professionals; the term 'witch-hunt', used to describe the search for professional culprits when an old person is found dead or a child in care is killed, symbolizes this attitude dramatically and clearly. The public do not wish the old people punished, in the sense in which that word is used today, but many people do want them 'put away', or in their terms 'cared for', to alleviate guilt and reduce anxiety.

The community physician's dilemma

These are the factors that the community physician has to bear in mind. But his basic dilemma is relatively simple: should he, or should he not, apply for an order for removal?

The first step is to decide whether or not removal is necessary; for in many cases it is possible to find a technical alternative to removal, thus freeing one from the ethical dilemma. If the problem is primarily environmental, with the old person living in 'insanitary conditions' or in conditions which are likely to cause an 'injury to the health of, or serious nuisance to, other persons', it is not necessary to remove the old person from his environment. In all the cases in which I have been involved it has been possible to improve the environment in which the old person is living. For the Public Health Act gives the community physician power, in co-operation with his colleagues in environmental health, to deal with flea-infested cats and dogs, clear accumulations of animal excreta, destroy soiled clothing and bedding, clean up filthy conditions in which rats are breeding, unblock toilets that are overflowing, clear blocked sewers, and remove accumulations of rubbish or rotting food. Sometimes the old person is very distressed by this type of intervention, and it is not one that is undertaken lightly. But if the old person is putting other people at risk then the ethical issue is clear-cut; the law can be invoked to fulfil its traditional purpose, namely the protection of the individual from harm by others, in this case harm from the old person who is living in insanitary conditions. This is the kind of intervention that is sanctioned by John Stuart Mill's famous principle that 'the sole end for which mankind are warranted, individually or collectively, in interfering with the liberty of action of any of their number is self-protection'.[15]

Secondly, it is essential to consider whether the old person can benefit only if he is removed from his dwelling or whether it is possible to provide a similar, or even greater, benefit by intervening in his own home. One's options are, of course, limited if the old person is not only refusing admission to hospital but also refuses to have domiciliary services such as home help or district nursing:

Miss S. lived alone in a semi-detached house and kept herself to herself. She visited the GP from time to time but had insisted that she was not in need of any help from the domiciliary services. The general practitioner was called to see her late one night in December and saw her lying in bed unable to open the door and obviously in need of some care and attention, for the house was very cold. It might have been possible to keep her in her own home by organizing district nursing and home help, but she adamantly refused to discuss the possibility of care in her own home. She was therefore compulsorily admitted to hospital, in spite of the fact that she did not require any treatment that could not have been given her in her own home.

If the person is willing to accept domiciliary care and if she has the type of problem that allows her to be dealt with at home, the community physician may face a different dilemma. For the extent to which it is possible to care for someone in their own home is a function not only of the nature of their problem; it is a function also of the resources that are available. If one were able to provide an old person suffering from pneumonia with one or two nurses right round the clock, then care at home would frequently be feasible. Given that resources are limited, however, and have to be spread thinly, it is not possible in practice to provide a person with two skilled nurses round the clock in their own home. In any case, the community physician knows full well that even if he were to press very hard for this level of domiciliary service and succeed in getting it, it would not be the ratepayers and taxpayers that paid for it; it would be other elderly people, whose services would have to be reduced to provide intensive care for this one individual. This would inevitably mean that other elderly people would have to go into institutional care sooner than would otherwise have been necessary, had not this one very assertive elderly person (or elderly person championed by a very assertive community physician) successfully demanded the intensive care in her own home instead of going into hospital when she had reached the conventional limits of domiciliary care. The community physician has, therefore, like all other professionals, to act as a rationer of resources; and when he tells an elderly person that it is not possible for her to be looked after in her own home, what he often means is that it is not possible to look after her in her own home with the amount of resources that are currently available, without creating inequities: without, that is, being unfair to his other clients.

Even if the old person cannot be looked after in her own home, the decision to apply for an order for compulsory removal is still a difficult one to take. The decision that admission is necessary is usually based on the need for specialist treatment; but, as I emphasized above, the order for compulsory removal does not confer the right to treat if the elderly person withholds her consent after admission. This has not been a common problem in practice, but a more difficult problem arises from the fact that the relocation of an elderly person itself carries an element of risk.

In 1976 the *British Medical Journal* published an article with the provocative title, 'Slow euthanasia or—"she will be better off in hospital"',[16] which received considerable publicity. There are, in fact, a number of detailed studies demonstrating the adverse effects of relocation.[17] It has been shown that both morbidity and mortality may be increased by uprooting elderly people from one environment and placing them in another that is supposedly more beneficial. Just how likely it is that removal will have an adverse effect depends on a number of factors. But it is known that physical illness, depression, and feelings of hopelessness are all associated with a higher probability that harmful consequences will follow if an old person is moved against her will; whereas these, ironically, are the very factors which usually give rise to the request for compulsory removal. The community physician therefore has to bear in mind not only the possible benefits of a move but also the possible harm that such a move may entail.

The question of competence

Where the community physician judges that an elderly person is incompetent, what he must try to do is act in a way that the person would herself, in her competent state, have approved of—would indeed approve of if, as lawyers sometimes say, she were to be granted a 'moment of lucidity'. This may be very difficult, if the community physician is given no information about her beliefs and attitudes before confusion set in.

Mrs S. had been widowed for many years. She lived in a flat above a church hall and for a number of years had been a conscientious caretaker, able both to look after herself and to help others. She developed both dementia and physical illness and after one admission to hospital her intellectual impairment became markedly worse. She was discharged to her flat, where she spent most of her time sitting in the kitchen neither eating the meals on wheels that were brought to her nor even drinking the tea that was poured out and left by her side. She was not completely immobile, however; for she used to go outside and wander in the road, looking for a cat that had been dead for three years. This behaviour continued until cold weather set in. She was obviously at serious risk, because she was found at two in the morning during a freezing night, wandering about dressed only in blouse and skirt calling for her cat.

She was compulsorily admitted to hospital and then transferred to an old-people's home. She said that she would like to go back home; but the church, on the advice of the health and social services, stated that they required her flat for other workers in the church. This was true, but to spare her feelings they omitted to say that they were afraid of her setting fire to her flat, the church hall, or the vicarage. She therefore continued to live in the old-people's home.

This woman had dementia, but the psychiatrist had decided that she could not be considered insane and therefore could not be removed using the Mental Health Act. The community physician therefore ruled her incompetent and obtained an order for her removal using the National Assistance Act.

The community physician is faced with a different problem if the person is not so obviously incompetent. Let us consider the case of Mr T.

Mr T. had recently retired. He lived alone in a room near the city centre and spent his days walking in the streets, sitting in the public library, and seeing friends. He was admitted to hospital for a bleeding ulcer, had an operation, and was then discharged, weak and anaemic. Unfortunately, he fell and twisted his knee and therefore became confined to his bed in his room. Because the meals-on-wheels service was unable to get into the multi-occupied house in which he lived, nobody knew that he was unable to get up until his landlord called his GP three weeks later, by which time his mattress and bedding were soaked with three weeks' accumulated urine and faeces.

His soiled bedding was then destroyed, he was washed and fed and made much more comfortable in bed; but his knee failed to improve, and he was obviously developing pneumonia in one lung. He said he did not want to die and that his wish was to get fit enough to walk about town again, but he still refused to go into hospital.

This man did not show any evidence of dementia, nor did he show any evidence of being confused as a result of his physical illness. Should a man like this be considered to be competent but misguided and therefore be removed by the community physician because he is making a wrong decision? Or should he be considered to be incompetent by virtue of the fact that he is making an illogical decision in wishing to remain active but refusing to go to hospital, which is the only means that would enable him to regain his previous level of activity? I was unable to work out the precise reasons for my action on that hot Sunday afternoon in his small cramped room; but I decided to remove him compulsorily. He told me that he did not think it was right. I replied that it might or might not be right, but that I considered it to be legal. He was admitted to hospital, made a good recovery, and was discharged to a hostel where he occupied a pleasant single room. When interviewed after discharge he was asked why he had kept refusing admission. He replied that he had simply kept telling himself that things could be worse.

The dilemma is even more dramatic when the person has a life-threatening illness, is incompetent by virtue of confusion or unconsciousness, and where there is a treatment for that illness that can be given only in hospital. In such cases the community physician has to decide whether the person's illness should be accepted as being a terminal illness or whether it should be considered to be a treatable or potentially curable disorder. This type of case is particularly difficult when the life-threatening illness is itself responsible for the confusion, a common occurrence in old age, when diseases such as pneumonia and congestive cardiac failure frequently cause confusion in addition to their physical signs and symptoms. In such cases the doctor has to rely on the reports of other people regarding the person's previous wishes and preferences; and it is sometimes very difficult to get an accurate account of the individual's beliefs and attitudes before the onset of the illness. Where the individual is known to have a severe degree of dementia, the problems of the professionals are obvious; for it is rare in this country for the elderly person to leave instructions that can help the professionals attending her when she develops dementia and an acute severe illness. In the United States, however, it has become common for elderly people to write 'living wills' setting out their views about the most appropriate way to manage severe life-threatening illness should they be incompetent to make a decision themselves. These living wills have been interpreted differently from State to State. In some States the medical profession has been strongly advised that it cannot assume that a living will could be taken as a legal instruction in a court of law if, for example, relatives were to sue a doctor who had omitted to treat an old person with pneumonia because she had said in her living will that she did not want to be given life-saving treatment were she to have developed dementia in the interim.

In the United Kingdom few people have taken this formal step. Perhaps because the population is less prone to litigation than in the United States, doctors intervene less in old age. In this country many doctors will not use antibiotics in the treatment of pneumonia, if the patient has dementia, although they and their nursing colleagues will take steps to ensure that the patient is well cared for, for example by being given adequate fluid. The doctor in this situation is making his decision within the ethical context defined by the values and attitudes of the society in which he is working.

Similar problems arise when the old person is known to have been opposed to any form of intervention before the onset of the disease that caused her confusional state. In such cases the community physician has to weigh up a number of factors, most notably the expressed wishes of the old person, her behaviour in the past when help was offered her, the likely course of events if her disorder is not treated, and the potential benefits of treatment.

The future of Section 47

Some people have argued that Section 47 should be repealed, on the ground that it represents an indefensible assault on the liberty of the individual.

My opinion is that, although Section 47 is certainly used to remove elderly people from their own homes, it can nevertheless be seen as a means of defending the rights of elderly people to live on in their own homes, when they are at risk or neglecting themselves. I base my opinion on two principal arguments. The first is that the repeal of Section 47 would not mean that large numbers of elderly people would be allowed to remain at home who are at present being compulsorily admitted to institutions. No, what would happen is what happens at the moment in those parts of the country in which the community physicians are known to be adamantly opposed to Section 47, or what happens when a community physician is unobtainable: the old person is simply coerced, deceived, or drugged in order to achieve an admission. As with the Mental Health Act, it is very important that we do not equate informal admissions, namely those that take place without legal powers being invoked, with voluntary admissions. In many parts of the country elderly people are admitted to, or kept in, institutions without the use of Section 47 who can certainly not be said to be voluntary patients who are willingly there as a result of decisions freely made. My second argument is that I would see Section 47 not so much as a means of infringing the liberty of individual elderly people, but, properly used with the support of magistrates determined to question the professionals concerned, as a means of controlling the liberty of professionals to act as they wish without recourse to the law.

The law is not simply a set of instruments; it is an expression of the values prevailing within society. The value expressed by Section 47 is that it is sometimes, albeit rarely, right for an individual's decisions to be overruled in his own interests. This is not, after all, an uncommon type of intervention. The law that compels a motorcyclist (unless he happens to be a Sikh) to wear a crash helmet, the law that requires motorists and front-seat passengers to wear seat-belts, and the law that makes it impossible to obtain certain medicines without a doctor's prescription, all have, in part, a paternalistic motive of this kind. They express the precept that, while it is an important value that people should be left free to make their own decisions, where others do not stand to be harmed thereby, this is not, *pace* Mill, an absolute value. Individual autonomy may sometimes be legitimately overridden for a person's own good, where the infringement of liberty is small as compared to the risk of harm if the individual is left to his own devices. What raises passions, where Section 47 is concerned, is the fact that old people are involved and the fact that the power rests largely with the discretion of a small number of individuals. But there is not, in my experience, any widespread evidence of this power being abused. So I should not be in favour of repealing the law.

There is, however, a case for amending it. If Section 47 is to remain an effective means of protecting individual elderly people from paternalistic relatives and professionals, and not to become merely a tool for the latter, its use should be more clearly monitored than it is at present. Unlike the compulsory removals made using the powers of the Mental Health Act, there is no requirement to notify the Department of Health and Social Security of the number of times the powers granted by Section 47 are used; thus there are no means of comparing the use made of the powers in different parts of the country. Similarly, no mechanism exists for scrutinizing the effects of compulsory removal. It seems to me that a system of review would provide the best safeguard against abuse. The decision to remove or not to remove has to be left to the discretion of the individual magistrate, guided by the professionals involved, and it would not be feasible to attempt to draw up a set of guidelines or conditions to cover all the varied circumstances that one encounters. Nevertheless it is highly desirable that doctor and magistrate should be made subject to the kind of accountability that a system of review would introduce.

5 AUTONOMY AND CONSENT

RAANAN GILLON

One of the commonest categories of medico-moral problems arises from conflict between the desire to do what is considered to be in the best interests of the patient and a desire to do what the patient says he wants (or may say he wants if given the opportunity to discuss the alternatives). Ultimately the conflict is between, on the one hand, beneficence, the principle that one should do good, and/or non-maleficence, the principle that one should not do harm (the Hippocratic principle *primum non nocere*); and on the other hand, the principle that one should respect people's autonomy. In this paper I shall discuss this conflict first by outlining what autonomy is, then by describing the principle of respect for autonomy and two disparate philosophical defences of it. Next I shall assess certain counter-arguments favouring paternalism, and finally I shall briefly consider cases where autonomy may be claimed either not to exist at all, or not to exist to an extent sufficient to be demanding of respect.

Consider three cases where respect for autonomy may have unpleasant, perhaps fatal results:

An old man has a malignant cancer with very poor prognosis. Among the options which standardly exist are palliative treatment with an acceptance that attempts to cure are extremely unlikely to succeed, and unpleasant, potentially lethal, chemotherapy, with or without radiotherapy, which none the less has some (remote) prospect of cure. Should either course of action be instituted without informing the patient of his condition and the available options, and without obtaining his informed consent?

A Jehovah's Witness is likely to die unless he is given a blood transfusion during a major surgical procedure. On religious grounds he has emphatically rejected the use of blood even if it is needed to save his life. Should his life be saved if the use of blood is the only way of doing so?

Until the 1970s it was British government policy to force-feed prisoners on hunger strike, with prison doctors doing the force-feeding in the prison hospital. A change in policy prohibited force-feeding, but on occasions when the prisoner has become comatose the relatives' request to institute artificial feeding has been met despite explicit instructions from the prisoner beforehand that he was to be left to starve to death if his political demands were not complied with. Should hunger-striking prisoners' lives be saved against their will?

The concept of autonomy

So what is autonomy? Essentially, autonomy is the capacity to think, decide, and act on the basis of such thought and decision, freely and independently and without, as it says in the passport, 'let or hindrance'. In the sphere of action, it is important to distinguish between, on the one hand, freedom, liberty, licence, or simply doing what one wants to do, and on the other hand acting autonomously, which may also be doing what one wants to do but on the basis of thought or reasoning. Animals are not said to have autonomy, but they may be perfectly 'free'—at liberty—in the sense that they are not constrained, for example, by cages, drugs, or having their wings pulled off by little boys. Autonomy is a subclass of freedom or liberty, but not all freedom or liberty is autonomy. The concept of autonomy is necessarily connected with the exercise of what Aristotle called man's specific attribute, rationality.

Autonomy is sometimes subdivided into autonomy of action, autonomy of will, and autonomy of thought. Autonomy of thought embraces the wide range of intellectual activities that are called 'thinking for oneself', including making decisions, believing things, having aesthetic preferences, and making moral assessments. Autonomy of will (or perhaps autonomy of intention) is the freedom to decide to do things on the basis of one's deliberations. Although the idea of 'the will' went into a phase of philosophical disrepute, it currently seems to be undergoing some sort of a rehabilitation.[1] For the ordinary man in the street and his doctor there is not much doubt that there is a human capacity corresponding to the idea of will-power—to the idea, for instance, that one can decide not to eat that second cream cake despite a powerful desire to do so. Equally, there is little doubt that some people have more of this autonomy of will than others do and that it may be diminished by disease or chemical agents. The patient, all of whose voluntary muscles are paralysed by curariforms but whose anaesthetist has forgotten the nitrous oxide, who tries in vain to stop the surgeon cutting him, is perhaps a paradigm of a person whose autonomy of thought and will are active but whose autonomy of action is for the time being completely absent. For autonomy of action is the freedom to act on the basis of one's autonomous thought and will. It should be noted that specific actions may be autonomous even though they are not the immediate or direct result of a thought process at all. One may drive to work perfectly autonomously without thinking what one is doing—one has put oneself, as it were, into autodrive. The point is, however, that one has decided on the basis of reasoning to do so and one's actions are, at any stage, responsive to reasoning; one may, for example, suddenly remember leaving the iron on and decide to turn back.[2] Autonomy of thought, of will (or intention), and of action requires some basis in reasoning.

John Benson, Professor of Philosophy at Lancaster University, in a stimulating paper on autonomy, describes it as a state of character manifesting reliance on one's own powers in acting, choosing, and forming opinions.[3] Seeing it as a virtue, he suggests, in Aristotelian vein, that it is a mean between, on the one hand, the deficiency of heteronomy, in which one is excessively influenced by others, for example by being credulous, gullible, compliant, passive, submissive, overdependent, or servile; and, on the other hand, the excess of arrogant self-sufficiency or even solipsism (acting as though one were the sole inhabitant of the moral universe). I do not accept that autonomy is a virtue. Rather it is a prerequisite, as I see it, for all the virtues, in that all virtues if they are to be virtues must, it seems to me, be based on actions stemming from deliberated choice—that is, they must be autonomous actions. (That, I take it, is why the concept of virtue has only a marginal application to non-human, non-rational animals.) Whether this is accepted or not, however, we can surely agree with Benson that autonomy is a characteristic possessed by people in varying degrees.

The principle of autonomy

The concept of autonomy must be distinguished from what is often known as the principle of autonomy, which is essentially the moral requirement to respect other people's autonomy. In practice, everyone accepts this principle to some extent: we all want our own autonomy respected (who would accept arbitrary imprisonment without even a *feeling* of moral outrage?) and we are all prepared to accept that we ought to respect the autonomy of at least some others in at least some circumstances. In the case of autonomy of action, however, the need for some restriction on respect for the autonomy of others is obvious; otherwise we should be morally required to respect any deliberated course of action no matter how horrible the consequences might be for others. Two great philosophers, one a founding father of utilitarianism, the other an exemplar of deontological (duty-based) ethical theorists, both argued vigorously for the moral importance of respecting people's autonomy; and both offered restrictions which, although expressed very differently, have, perhaps, some similarities. John Stuart Mill argued that respect for another's autonomy was required in so far as such respect did not result in harm to others and in so far as the people thus respected possessed a fairly basic level of maturity (a capability 'of being improved by free and equal discussion').[4] Immanuel Kant argued that both autonomy and respect for the autonomy of others were necessary features of any rational agent in so far as their exercise conformed to the 'categorical imperative'. Let me offer very brief, very rough, and oversimplified accounts of their respective claims.

Kant's metaphysics divides what exists into two great realms, the intelligible or 'noumenal' world—the world of reason—and the phenomenal world, the world of sense perception. What exists in both these realms works in accordance with universal laws.[5] A rational being has 'the power to act in accordance with his idea of laws'. Non-rational beings, however, are acted upon, and their behaviour is causally necessitated or determined by causes outside themselves. Human beings are an amalgam of the rational and the non-rational; it is the will that links these aspects of man, enabling him to use his reason to produce effects on the non-rational world, including the non-rational aspects of himself. 'Will is a kind of causality belonging to living beings so far as they are rational. Freedom would then be the property this causality has of being able to work independently of determination by alien causes.' In so far as human beings are ruled by forces other than their own will, including the 'impulsions of animal nature', they act heteronomously. In so far as they are rational agents they are ruled by their own will and are thus autonomous. Now, as we have seen, whatever exists in either sphere works according to universal laws and Kant argues that there is only one objective moral law for the autonomous will, though it may be presented in several ways. This is his famous 'categorical imperative' that requires us to 'act only on that maxim through which you can at the same time will that it should become a universal law'. His argument for this is that all objective moral laws necessarily apply to all rational agents and therefore no maxim (principle on which we in fact act) *could* be consistent with such objective moral laws unless the maxim could consistently be willed by the agent to be a universal law applying to all rational agents. The inherent dignity of any person (by which Kant means any rational being) lies in his ability not merely to confirm to the moral law, but to choose to do so, to accept the law for himself (as distinct, for instance, from being forced by someone else to obey it, which is just as heteronomous as allowing one's 'animal impulsions' to make one behave contrary to the moral law).

It is in this way that people can be both subject to universal moral laws and yet at the same time be authors of those laws, in that they have subjected themselves willingly to them. Rational beings necessarily have wills, according to Kant, and thus are by their nature ends in themselves as distinct from mere means; and this is true both objectively and subjectively, in that this is how men necessarily conceive of their own existence. Any application of the categorical imperative must recognize that fact. From this Kant derives (or some would say purports to derive) his other formulations of the categorical imperative: 'Act in such a way that you always treat humanity, whether in your own person or in the person of any other, never simply as a means but always at the same time as an end' and 'a rational being must always regard himself as making laws in a kingdom of ends', where a kingdom of ends is a 'systematic union of different rational beings under common laws'.

For Kant, then, self-rule—autonomy—is a fundamental and logically necessary feature of being a rational agent: 'Autonomy is therefore the ground of the dignity of human nature and of every rational nature.'

J. S. Mill also argued for the moral requirement to respect the autonomy of others, supporting this claim (as does Oxford's Professor R. M. Hare[6]) on the utilitarian grounds that such respect (which should, according to Mill, 'govern absolutely the dealings of society with the individual in the way of compulsion and control'[7]) would maximize human welfare. Mill has traditionally been pilloried for attempting to square the circle in endorsing both an absolute principle of respect for liberty (by which he clearly means autonomy) and utilitarianism; but in a recent book, the Oxford philosopher John Gray puts up a good case for Mill's consistency here.[8] Gray points out that Mill, while insisting that the principle of utility is 'the ultimate appeal on all ethical questions', also stresses that it must be utility understood 'in the largest sense grounded on the permanent interests of a man as a progressive being'.[9] Thus understood, the principle of utility may be seen as having the principle of respect for autonomy as a corollary. This is because human happiness is constituted, in part, by the exercise of individual autonomy. Moreover, each person exercises his autonomy differently, and thus his happiness (in the broad Aristotelian sense of *eudaimonia* or flourishing), which partially depends upon his fulfilment of the demands of his own nature, will also be different. Maximal respect for the exercise of individual autonomy (so far as this does not harm others) is thus a precondition for the utilitarian objective of maximizing human welfare.[10] It is in this context that I now quote Mill's introductory assertion in *On Liberty*:

The object of this Essay is to assert one very simple principle, as entitled to govern absolutely the dealings of society with the individual in the way of compulsion and control . . . That principle is, that the sole end for which mankind are warranted, individually or collectively, in interfering with the liberty of action of any of their number, is self-protection. That the only purpose for which power can rightfully be exercised over any member of a civilized community, against his will, is to prevent harm to others. His own good, either physical or moral, is not a sufficient warrant.[11]

To summarize the argument thus far: autonomy is the capacity to think, to decide, and to act on the basis of such thought and decision. Respect for autonomy is the moral principle that people should have their autonomy respected to the extent that such respect is consistent with respect for the autonomy of others (and I have not gone into the problems surrounding this condition). Part of what such respect for autonomy implies, in practical terms, is not interfering with people without their consent— not imposing interference on people. Mill defends this moral principle on the utilitarian grounds that such respect for autonomy furthers human welfare. Kant defends it on the grounds that rational agents—and therefore men in so far as they are, and are acting as, rational agents—necessarily recognize the requirement to treat people as ends in themselves—as self-ruling or autonomous—and not merely as means.

I am not sure that I accept the Kantian argument that all rational agents *necessarily* recognize the moral obligation to respect others as autonomous, as ends in themselves. Perhaps it depends on the sense of necessity involved. But there can be little doubt that whenever one does not recognize and respect another's autonomy, then one is necessarily not treating him as (allowing him to be) a rational agent; for rational agency by definition requires autonomy. (It is action grounded in one's deliberation and decision.) Thus whenever, for example, one imposes decisions upon people without consulting them, let alone against their will, whether or not these decisions are designed to be beneficial, one is treating them as things or as animals or as children, but not as rational agents, not as ends in themselves.

Medical paternalism

But the obvious question is: Why *should* we always treat other people as rational agents, as ends in themselves, rather than merely as means to an end? Many would argue, on the contrary, that sometimes when we want to help people, especially in the context of medical care, we are obliged to treat them merely as means—means to their own recovery, for example. The model usually offered is that of the relationship between a father and his infant, the model of benevolent paternalism (or parentalism, as some Californians now insist on saying).

Imagine that your six-year-old son is afflicted by acute leukaemia and your colleague, the paediatric oncologist, tells you that aggressive chemotherapy has a good chance, say a 70 per cent five-year survival rate, of curing the condition. Considerable morbidity may result as each course of treatment is given, with nausea and vomiting, anxiety, hair loss, increased risk of infection, excessive marrow inhibition, and probable permanent sterility. What should you, his doctor parent, do? Should you discuss the issues with the child, describe the alternative courses of action and their pros and cons (including the almost inevitable death that will follow if treatment is not undertaken) and then help him to come to his own decision? Of course not. You and your spouse weigh up these factors and decide on the best course of action, making it as easy as possible for the child to bear (which will doubtless involve some truth-telling, some explanation, but perhaps also evasions, deceit, and lies as well, and no real options or choice-making, no difficult decisions for the child to make). Regardless of whether the child accepts your decision, you authorize its implementation, behaving as comfortingly and supportively as you can, knowing that you have made what you believe to be the best available choice in the best interests of your child. That is an example of paternalism.[12] Can there really be any valid criticisms to be levelled at that? Of course not (though I do not doubt that there are some rabid libertarians—even more rabid than I, that is—who would find it offensively paternalistic). It is ethically more problematic, however, when such behaviour is meted out not to one's six-year-old child but to one's patients, of all ages. Yet undoubtedly such attitudes of benevolent paternalism have, for at least 2,500 years, characterized, to a greater or lesser extent, the behaviour of the vast majority of doctors towards their patients; and I do not think many would deny that they still permeate much of contemporary medical practice.

Various (supposed) justifications underlie the practice of medical paternalism. The most important is that medical ethics is often supposed to require it: the Hippocratic Oath can be understood as requiring it when it says 'I will prescribe regimen for the good of my patients according to my ability and judgement and never do harm to anyone.' This can be understood to mean that it is the doctor's responsibility to do what, to the best of his judgement and ability, he can do in the best interests of his patient, regardless of whether the patient agrees with this judgement of where his best interests lie, regardless of whether the patient has given explicit consent to the action(s) proposed, and regardless of whether the patient knows the likely consequences and the available alternatives.

Put like that the duty sounds less obviously attractive; but put in terms of real-life situations with patients terrified by their diseases, perhaps suffering great pain and other unpleasant symptoms such as breathlessness, and being utterly bewildered, then it becomes far more plausible to think, if one is that patient's doctor or relative, that the last thing one should do is add to his misery and uncertainty by telling him the results of his biopsy or the risk of the treatment or whatever other nasty bits of information one has up one's sleeve. More plausible indeed, but not necessarily right.

First, even if one accepts the consequentialist claim that all that matters, morally speaking, is that one do the best one can for one's patient's health and to minimize his suffering, it is not clear that this end is furthered by evasions, deceit, and downright lies. Of course such behaviour (the hearty slap on the back, 'Well we're not magicians of course, old boy, but we'll do our best for you—you can rest assured of that—and we have had some *excellent* results . . .') greatly reduces the anguish for the doctors: honest discussions concerning their condition and prospects with people who have fatal diseases are emotionally very demanding, as is the necessary follow-up; it is far less difficult to 'look on the bright side'. But, as Roger Higgs argues in a subsequent chapter (see below, pp. 187–202), the assumption that people with serious or fatal conditions are, in general, happier if they are deceived about them is highly suspect. What is more, it is usually only the patient who is deceived, while a relative or relatives are told the truth; the deceit that this imposes on the family can itself provoke considerable distress (not to mention the breaking of the normal principle of medical confidentiality and *its* effects). Finally, fatally ill people treated thus frequently discover before they die that they have been deceived by their doctors and their families.[13] What a way to go! Some patients, it is true, want their doctors to shield them from any unpleasant information and to take over decision-making on all fronts concerning their illness. My point is that not all do. Moreover it requires some skill, time, and effort to find out what the patient really does want; too often it is merely assumed that the patient 'doesn't want to know'.

The second line of justification of paternalistic behaviour is that patients are not capable of making decisions about medical problems: they are too ignorant medically speaking. Such knowledge as they do have is too partial, in both senses of the word. Because of this they are unlikely to be able to understand what is going on even if it is explained to them. Therefore they are likely to make worse decisions than the doctor would. Even if one were to accept that 'best decisions' are the sole or overriding moral determinant in such cases, it is worth distinguishing the sorts of decisions which doctors might be expected to make better than their patients from the sorts of decisions where there is little or no reason to expect this to be the case. In the technical area for which they have been specially and extensively trained there is little doubt that a doctor will make a more probably correct (and hence in that sense better) decision than his medically ignorant patient. Thus the doctor who advises his patient that to continue with her pregnancy would, because of her coexisting medical conditions, be from her point of view a markedly more dangerous course of action than to have a termination, and that therefore a termination would be better, may be giving a medically sound piece of advice based on his medical knowledge. But for him to insist or even suggest that a termination would be better in some moral sense would be for him to step outside his realm of competence: he is no better trained professionally to make that kind of moral assessment than is his patient. And even if he were, many would object that it is not the doctor's role even to advise on his patient's moral decisions, let alone make them for her.

The counter-argument just offered meets the paternalist on his own ground in accepting that there are some areas, notably the technical medical areas, in which doctors may be expected to make better decisions than their patients. But it points out that there still remain other areas, notably the moral area, in which there is little reason to expect them to do so. A further matter on which it is doubtful whether doctors are qualified or likely to make better decisions than their patients concerns what course of action can be expected to produce most happiness or least unhappiness, all things considered (the utilitarian calculus). Some doctors believe, for example, that, in the case of severely handicapped new-born infants, it is up to them to 'shoulder the burden', assess what course of action is going to produce the greatest benefit all things considered, and then implement it. As one doctor has put it, 'In the end it is usually the doctor who has to decide the issue. It is . . . cruel to ask the parents whether they want their child to live or die.'[14] But as Buchanan points out, if a doctor is going to undertake to assess which of various available courses of action (including, say, letting die on the one hand, and surgery and other intensive therapy on the other) is most probably going to produce the greatest happiness all things considered, he is going to have to consider an awful lot of factors.[15]

[T]he physician must first make intrapersonal comparisons of harm and benefit of each member of the family, if the information is divulged. Then he must somehow coalesce these various intrapersonal net harm judgments into an estimate of total net harm which divulging the information will do to the family as a whole. Then he must make similar intrapersonal and interpersonal net harm judgments about the results of not telling the truth. Finally, he must compare these totals and determine which course of action will minimise harm to the family as a whole.[16]

Buchanan makes a similar analysis for the doctor who tries seriously to assess whether it would be best all things considered to tell a dying patient the truth. After demonstrating the complexity of any such analysis and its necessarily morally evaluative components, Buchanan concludes:

once the complexity of these judgments is appreciated and once their evaluative character is understood it is implausible to hold that the physician is in a better position to make them than the patient or his family. The failure to ask what sorts of harm/benefit judgments may properly be made by the physician in his capacity as a physician is a fundamental feature of medical paternalism.[17]

Of course such assessments—moral assessments and preference assessments—are difficult for anybody to make. But there is no prima facie reason to suppose that doctors make them better than their patients. Even in the case of technical medical assessments the argument from patient ignorance is highly suspect, for there exist plenty of doctors who are able to explain technical medical issues to their patients' satisfaction. Perhaps those who cannot, rather than arguing that it cannot be done, might consider (a) handing over the task to someone who can, and/or (b) obtaining some simple postgraduate training in more effective communication with their patient. Better late than never.

All these counter-arguments try to meet the defence of paternalism on its own ground by accepting its assumption that achieving the outcome which produces greatest happiness, either for the patient alone or, in more complex cases, for his family, or even perhaps for society as a whole, is the only goal—the full-blown utilitarian position. Those who reject this objective of maximizing happiness as being sufficient for any adequate moral theory will argue that respect for certain other moral principles such as promise-keeping, truth-telling, avoiding deceit, and in general respect for the autonomy of others (which I believe underpins these other moral principles) should in any case act as constraints upon a simple utilitarianism or even replace it entirely. (One must add, however, that there are more complex types of utilitarianism, such as that favoured by Professor Hare,[18] which attempt to incorporate such principles.) Such pluralists will argue that even if it is true, in a particular case, that most sane, mature adults would, on reflection, agree that the doctor's decision is better than his patient's, all things considered—that the patient will do better, live longer, be cured more effectively, or whatever—still there remains a whole host of cases where the patient's autonomy must be respected, to the extent of allowing him or her to make the worse decision, even if this will result in his or her death. I earlier gave examples of the hunger-strikers and the Jehovah's Witnesses. A moving variant was offered in the *British Medical Journal* by Sir Richard Bayliss in his description of a Christian Scientist who, by rejecting the advice and treatment of orthodox medicine in favour of that of Christian Science, died for her beliefs.[19] (Her decision to return to the care of orthodox medicine came too late to save her life.) Few who do not share Christian Scientism can believe that she made a 'better' decision in relation to her health than that advised by her original doctor. But those of us who place a respect for individual autonomy very high in the moral hierarchy would not deny her the respect of allowing her to make such a decision, even though it is a disastrously worse decision, and even though it causes us great personal anguish to stand by and watch a person die unnecessarily.

Thus even if one accepts a consequentialist position (according to which it is only the outcome of an action that matters morally speaking), paternalism is a suspect stance; and respect for people's autonomy seems to rule it out in general.

Some qualifications

So, does all this respect for autonomy, which I have been defending, mean that people must never have decisions taken for them by others? In particular, in medical practice, does explicit and informed consent have to be obtained for each and every medical decision? I do not believe so. In the last part of this paper I shall outline why. Before doing so, however, let me mention in parentheses that 'informed consent' does not, in my view, mean a signature on a long and legalistic document outlining all possible risks and benefits of a proposed procedure. Rather than argue this here, I will content myself with referring you to an excellent paper on informed consent by the Chairman of the Australian Law Reform Commission.[20] The nub of informed consent involves giving the patient sufficient information for him to be able to make a reasonable decision.

The first qualification arises from the fact that people may autonomously decide to delegate medical decision-making to their doctors. For doctors to take medical decisions on behalf of their patients in such circumstances is clearly not to override a person's autonomy (though of course the important issue here is whether or not the patient has autonomously delegated such decision-making). People vary enormously in this respect and, especially when they are ill, very often want the doctor to take decisions for them, on the natural assumption that the doctor will do so in such a way as to maximize his patient's chances of a return to health, minimizing his risks in so doing. Provided patients genuinely wish their doctors to take just such decisions, no infringement of their autonomy is involved if a doctor accedes to this desire.

A second qualification is that illness can produce a dramatic diminution in a person's autonomy, a situation well described by Pellegrino.[21] Thus, depending on the severity of the patient's medical condition, the doctor may have to deal with a human being who is anything from totally unconscious to thoroughly autonomous. The problem of absent or very diminished autonomy is an enormous one and is vigorously debated. Suffice it to say here that two important principles should, I believe, inform assessments. The first is that, where the patient is unable to make his own decisions, the decision to be aimed at, so far as is possible, is the decision he would, were he able to make it, make for himself. In practical terms, and indeed in legal terms, the prima facie assumption must surely be that the patient's next of kin and/or loved ones are in the best position to ascertain these counter-factual wishes. This is not invariably the case, however, and it is always open to a doctor to apply to a court where he believes that the patient's own interests are being jeopardized or overridden by the next of kin. The second important principle concerns patients whose autonomy is diminished. Some have argued that in such cases the doctor's duty is to restore the patient's premorbid autonomy, even if this involves overriding such autonomy as the patient has left.[22] Clearly, in society in general, a minimal level of autonomy is required before a person is socially recognized and accepted as being an autonomous agent. In democratic societies, this level is a very basic one; once people attain it they are regarded as 'competent' and their autonomy is respected, however reduced it may be compared to that of many others in the society. I do not propose to discuss the justification for accepting such low levels of autonomy as grounding legal competence and the requirement for respect for autonomy; but it is difficult to see any justification for doctors to set a *higher* level of competence which their patients must manifest if their autonomy is to be respected.

If mere evidence of impairment of autonomy (or even of serious impairment) is to be used to justify compulsory intervention by others in order to increase people's autonomy then all standard concepts of respect for autonomy and respect for individual liberty will have taken on new, and to many somewhat sinister meanings.[23]

Given that the same level of competence above which a person's autonomy is not to be overridden is accepted for patients as for people in the rest of society, there still remains a host of very difficult problems concerning the determination of a person's actual level of autonomy, and therefore of his competence. This problem becomes particularly acute in the context of psychiatric disease. While I have suggested that society in general should determine the sort of levels of autonomy above which a person is to be considered competent, it seems sensible for society to delegate to experts the task of deciding whether such levels are attained in particular and doubtful cases; in the case of mental disease, for example, that task might be delegated to psychiatrists and psychologists specially trained and experienced in making such assessments. But a detailed treatment of these issues lies beyond the scope of this paper.[24]

6 WHICH SLOPES ARE SLIPPERY?

BERNARD WILLIAMS

In many ethical connections, including those in which the discussion concerns what the law should be, there is a well-known argument against allowing some practice that it leads to, or is at the top of, or is on, a slippery slope. The argument is of course often applied to matters of medical practice. If X is allowed, the argument goes, then there will be a *natural progression* to Y; and since the argument is intended as an objection to X, Y is presumably agreed to be objectionable, while X is not (though of course it may be objectionable to the proponent of the argument—the slippery slope may be only one of his objections to it). The central question that needs to be asked about such arguments is what is meant by a 'natural progression'. Before coming to that, however, we need to make one or two preliminary points. First, it is worth distinguishing two types of slippery-slope argument. The first type—the *horrible result* argument—objects, roughly speaking, to what is at the bottom of the slope. The second type objects to the fact that it is a slope: this may be called the *arbitrary result* argument.

An example of a *horrible result* argument is that sometimes used against *in vitro* fertilization of human ova, or at least against practices that are associated with that. IVF gives rise to extra fertilized ova, and experimentation is at least permitted, and perhaps required, on those ova. The period of time during which such experiments are allowed is limited, but (the argument goes) there is a natural progression to longer and longer such periods being permitted, until we arrive at the horrible result of experimentation on developed embryos.

All the arguments that I shall be considering use the idea that there is no point at which one can non-arbitrarily get off the slope once one has got on to it—that is what makes the slope slippery.

Arguments that belong to the first type that I have distinguished involve, in addition, the further idea that there is a clearly objectionable practice to which the slope leads.

The second type of argument, by contrast, relies merely on the point that after one has got on to the slope, subsequent discriminations will be arbitrary. Suppose that some tax relief or similar benefit is allowed to couples only if they are legally married. It is proposed that the benefit be extended to some couples who are not married. Someone might not object to the very idea of the relief being given to unmarried couples, but nevertheless argue that the only non-arbitrary line that could be drawn was between the married couples and the unmarried, and that as soon as any unmarried couple was allowed the benefit, there would be too many arbitrary discriminations to be made.

Not all cases in which a slippery slope comes into the discussion are genuinely slippery-slope arguments. Sometimes the slope is invoked in order to express some other ground of objection. This is sometimes the case with Catholic objections to abortion. If it is said that early abortion is on a slippery slope that ends in infanticide, this may be a way of expressing another objection, itself regarded as basic, to the effect that early abortion is an example of killing an innocent human being. The slippery-slope considerations are intended to make one see that point, but the point itself goes beyond them. (I shall briefly discuss that sort of argument at the end of this paper, and also the point that some arguments fail to make clear the ways in which they depend on slippery-slope considerations.) By contrast, someone might base an objection to abortion directly on the slippery-slope argument itself, without agreeing that all abortion consisted of killing an innocent human being. He or she might think that early abortion did not involve doing that, but that there was a natural progression to cases that did.

There is another distinction to be made—a particularly important one. If it is said, in the course of one of these arguments, that two different cases or practices, A and B, cannot appropriately be distinguished, one thing that this may mean is that a distinction between them cannot *reasonably* be defended. It may be said, for instance, that any criterion or principle that admits A must admit B. Alternatively, it might be said that even though some distinction between A and B can reasonably be defended (there is a decent argument for distinguishing them), they cannot *effectively* be distinguished, and, as a matter of social or psychological fact, if A is admitted, B will be. Both these ideas, of a reasonable distinction and of an effective one, are relative to the nature of the practices and purposes in question. There must be some difference between A and B for the discussion even to get going, but that difference (between two foetuses, one of which is a day older than the other, for instance) may be said not to be reasonable in relation to what is being discussed (abortion), or not to be effective, or both.

A reasonable distinction need not be an effective one. Consider first-personal cases of temptation and discipline (to which indeed social cases of the slippery slope are often assimilated). If someone is trying to regulate smoking or eating, it may well be that in terms of the effects that are to be controlled—ill health, obesity, and so on—the distinction between no cigarettes or chocolate biscuits a day, and one, is not significant, and certainly less significant than that between one a day and thirty; but nevertheless the distinction between none and one is effective, while that between one and thirty is not, just because none does not lead to one, but one does lead to thirty.

When one is considering cases in which policies are to be adopted socially, and not solely for one person, there are further reasons why a distinction which was reasonable in terms of the original issues may turn out not to be effective. It may be clear, for instance, that the original case will be diffusely and inaccurately perceived in society. Again, not everyone in society may share the original judgements of what was reasonable. There may be a consensus on not allowing X, but as soon as X is allowed, there may be no consensus on what further distinctions can be drawn, and this may predictably lead to the undesired result Y. In such cases, we can have distinctions which are reasonable but not effective. They are distinctions which are intrinsically reasonable merely in terms of the subject-matter, but if one tries to base policy on those distinctions, there are social factors which mean that it will not stick. In similar terms, there can be distinctions which will be effective but are not (otherwise) reasonable.

There are some special questions about the distinction between the reasonable and the effective when one is concerned with *arbitrary result* cases, as I have called them. These questions arise particularly where issues of justice are involved, and the agent is publicly answerable for the equitable character of what is done. It may be argued, for instance, that no exception should be made to a certain rule, even though the particular exception being proposed is perfectly reasonable in terms of the purpose of the rule and the nature of the particular exception: the argument being that one will not be able to distinguish reasonably between the many possible exceptions that may then be claimed or, again, that the distinctions involved could not effectively be justified to the public. This is of course the territory of the academics' friend, the Thin End of the Wedge, or what Keynes used to call the Principle of Equal Unfairness, that one should not do a good turn to one person, for fear that you might have to do one for someone else. There are, of course, cases in which this kind of argument is sound, but there are at least two ways in which it may fail. One is that the agents may be taking too narrow a view of what can count as a relevant distinction. Thus if somebody applies for a grant on grounds which are all right in themselves, it may not be much of an objection (though it is often heard) to say that if the grant is given, there will be no money for some other applicant with a similar claim: *being the first applicant* can itself be a relevant characteristic in such cases. Another way in which the argument can fail is that it may simply not be true that this exception or good turn will generate more demands for exceptions or good turns. The mere idea that there *could* be a row of claimants whose cases one could not distinguish cannot be enough to support this kind of slippery-slope argument.

But what does it mean to say that one cannot distinguish one case from another? A fundamental point here is that, in these applications of it as in many others, *indistinguishable from* is not a transitive relation: from the fact that A is indistinguishable from B and that B is indistinguishable from C, it does not follow that A is indistinguishable from C. This is familiar with regard to distinguishing colours by eye, but it applies equally to drawing reasonable distinctions among ways in which different cases are to be treated.

If indistinguishability in a given respect is made the basis of the application of a general term, a problem can notoriously arise, often discussed in terms of the paradox of the heap;[1] problems about slippery slopes are interestingly related to paradoxes of this sort. If a pile of n grains of sand constitutes a heap, it is plausible to say that so must a pile of $[n - 1]$ grains; but equally obviously you can find some number m such that a pile of m grains or less is not a heap. In general, suppose we have a range of objects which we can place in order, on the basis of some varying characteristic, so that each object in the series will differ from its immediate neighbours, in terms of this characteristic, by only a tiny amount. (Piles of sand ordered by the number of grains they contain would be merely one example of this.) Let the objects be numbered $0[1]$, $0[2]$, and so on, according to their position in the series. Now suppose there is some property, call it the property of being F (in the above example, being a heap), which relates to the above characteristic in such a way that apparently

(1) $0[1]$ is F.
(2) For any number n, if $0[n]$ is F, so is $0[n + 1]$ (in the heap case, so is $0[n - 1]$).
(3) For some number m, $0[m]$ is not F.

The problem then is that the conjunction of these three statements seems to be self-contradictory.

There are many ethical predicates that are vague in ways that invite the paradox. (Aristotle's doctrine of the Mean, indeed, taken strictly, implies that all expressions standing for virtues or vices display such vagueness.[2]) In some cases, so long as the structure within which judgements are being made is relatively informal, or contains a high degree of consensus, and it is not under pressure, we may be able to proceed as we proceed with many other vague predicates: we adopt the resource of what might be called *restricted judgement*, and make judgements that involve the predicate in question only in cases that either clearly display it, or clearly fail to do so. How precisely that resource deals with the paradox is another question; one way of understanding it might be that there is nothing in our practice to commit us to the assertion of the induction step (2) above, nor to its denial. However this may be, the practice at least keeps the paradox at bay.

If we consider the special case, however, of normative predicates, such as 'may reasonably be given a grant', 'may rightfully be aborted', and so on—a class which is particularly relevant to slippery-slope arguments—this resource is less likely to succeed. If a case presents itself at all, the practical question of what one should do cannot be avoided. So virtually the only circumstances in which the resource of restricted judgement remains available are those in which the cases that actually present themselves come from distinct parts of the range (as if, for example, requests for abortions obligingly only ever came very early or very late in pregnancy). One is not necessarily (as I pointed out earlier in connection with certain *arbitrary result* cases) compelled to make a decision for cases that never in practice arise.

There are, however, several factors that may upset that situation. One may not be that lucky with the cases (we shall consider shortly circumstances that make it unlikely that one will be lucky.) Moreover, it may well be that judgements are demanded about cases that have not actually presented themselves. This is likely to be so if the structure in which these decisions are being made is formal, public, and less consensual than those that typically sustain the resource of restricted judgement. In particular, it will be so if there is a requirement of publicity, and a declaration is demanded of what principle is being employed: a demand that may be made so that the practices can be understood and criticized, and so that people can have determinate expectations of how they might be affected by those practices. In these circumstances—and they are not confined to the use of the law, though that is an obvious example—the resource of restricted judgement will not do.

I mentioned that there were circumstances in which one was unlikely to remain lucky with the selection of cases that present themselves. These are the circumstances that most typically offer the conditions for a slippery-slope argument. It is particularly so when there is a precedent effect. Here, the fact that a given case has presented itself makes it likely that the next case will present itself, because there are people who have an interest in the next case being decided in the same way as the last, and it seems unreasonable that the next case, since it is indeed the next case in the spectrum, should not be decided in the same way as the last. There is more than one reason why this process is likely to be repeated. It is not merely that, at any given stage, there seems no adequate reason to refuse the next step. In addition, it may well be that when a number of steps has been taken, the original objections to the process, or to this degree of it, now seem misplaced. The cumulative process has itself altered perceptions of that process. It is a mechanism very like that in terms of which Nelson Goodman explained the fact that increasingly incompetent forgeries by van Meegeren were accepted as genuine Vermeers.[3] Each new one was compared to a reference class that contained the earlier ones, and it was only when all the forgeries were bracketed, and the latest ones compared to a class of Vermeers free from van Meegerens, that it became obvious how awful they were. It is often this kind of process that critics have in mind when they claim that allowing some process will lead to a slippery slope. It is a process that they see in terms of corruption or habituation, just as reformers may see it as a process of enlightenment or of inhibitions being lost.

When may one rightly appeal to a process of this kind, and what are the correct conclusions to be drawn from it? The first requirement—to repeat a point that has already been made—is that it should be probable in actual social fact that such a process will occur. That requires that there should be some motive for people to move from one step to the next. Those who favour conservative policies sometimes simply assume this, perhaps because they have in mind a model of social addiction: once started in some given direction, society has, like the incipient alcoholic, an irresistible urge to go progressively further down the same path. In some cases, there certainly are reasons for thinking that the process is likely to occur. Besides the sort of examples suggested up to now, where interested parties have the same motive in relation to later cases as such parties had with earlier cases, there is also the competitive or many-party situation, supposedly exemplified by the arms race,[4] in which each party has a reason to take the next step because some other party took the last step. The conditions for a slide can be fulfilled in various different ways, but one must try as best one may to find out whether in a given situation they will be fulfilled or not. Possible cases are not enough, and the situation must have some other feature which means that those cases have to be confronted.

Suppose it is plausible that there will be a slide, and that there will be, at each stage, pressure to take the next step. What follows from that? The slippery-slope argument concludes that one should not start, and that the first case (whatever exactly that may be) should not be allowed, on the ground that after the first step there is nowhere to stop. In terms of the paradox, the argument wants us not to let premiss (1) above be true. But there is an obvious alternative. Granted that we are now considering cases in which a definite rule or practice is needed, which can be applied to any case and does not rely on what I called earlier 'restricted judgement', we have the alternative of sharpening the normative predicate in question, and drawing a sharp line between cases that are allowed and cases that are not. In terms of the paradox, the effect will be that premiss (2), the induction step, is falsified: for some n, we shall have decided that F applies to $0[n]$ but not to $0[n + 1]$. We lay down a maximum length of pregnancy for abortion, a number of days during which experiments on a fertilized ovum are permitted, a minimum age for admission to certain sorts of films, and so on.

Is drawing a line in this way reasonable? Can it be effective? The answer to both these questions seems to me evidently to be 'Yes, sometimes', and as that unexciting reply suggests, there is not a great deal to be brought to deciding them beyond good sense and relevant information. It may be said that a line of this kind cannot possibly be reasonable since it has to be drawn between two adjacent cases in the range—that is to say, between two cases that were not different enough to distinguish. The answer is that they are indeed not different enough to distinguish, if that means that their characteristics, unsupported by anything else, would have led one to draw a line there. But it is, all the same, reasonable to draw a line there. That follows from the conjunction of three things. First, it is reasonable to distinguish in some way unacceptable cases from acceptable cases; secondly, the only way of doing that in these circumstances is to draw a sharp line; thirdly, it cannot be an objection to drawing the line just here that it would have been no worse to draw it somewhere else—if that were an objection, one could conclude, by cumulation, that one had no reason to draw it anywhere, a path that leads to the grave of Buridan's ass (which allegedly starved through indecision, when placed between two equally attractive bales of hay). In practice, of course, the point at which the line is drawn is often chosen because it is salient in some way. Moreover, and significantly, it is rarely set directly in terms of the characteristic that the argument is about (development of a foetus, emotional maturity of a film-goer), but is based rather on something else (a date, an age) which can be clearly established and is roughly correlated with the relevant characteristics. This makes it all the clearer that it is not the precise merits of one rather than another step in the range that is in question when the line is drawn.

The proposed line may be unreasonable on some other grounds, but it is not so merely because it is this kind of line. Whether it will be effective is another question. If it is less effective than the alternative of allowing no cases at all, that will be because of special circumstances, such as those in which there is a consensus for allowing no cases, if that is all that can be achieved, but no consensus for anything else. Equally familiar, on the other hand, is the situation in which there is a consensus for allowing something rather than nothing, and a further consensus gradually emerges about what is to be allowed—formed, perhaps, as a result of action taken in advance of any consensus.

On this account, the slippery-slope argument, properly understood, is very largely an empirical, consequentialist, argument. It does of course assume certain evaluations, for instance about the horrible result (in that version of the argument) indeed being horrible. It also has to make assumptions about what decisions are demanded; on the question, for instance, whether it would be equitable, as well as possible, to rely on the resources of restricted judgement. It has to make judgements about what would be a reasonable distinction, in the light both of the subject-matter considered in itself and of the possible value of drawing a sharp line somewhere, in the way that we have just examined. But after all that, the argument is only about what sort of social practice will in fact follow from adopting what kind of rule.

Some people feel that the argument goes deeper than this account suggests, and that it relates to some basic moral requirements on policy. They resist the idea, in very serious matters, of basing policy on 'sharpening' a predicate which otherwise invites a slippery-slope argument (as we might, for example, arbitrarily define 'heap of sand' to mean 'pile of sand containing over ten thousand grains'). They think that fundamental issues cannot turn on matters of degree, or on an 'arbitrary' resolution of those matters. They may feel that real moral indistinguishability must be transitive, so that if a distinction is to be made, it should be based on some non-scalar, relevant difference. On this view of things, it is incomprehensible that one course of action might be right (acceptable, tolerable) and another wrong (unacceptable, intolerable) *simply* because they differed in the degree to which they possessed some scalar characteristic. The natural expression of this view is to try to base the distinctions relevant to these important matters on properties which do not admit of degrees—as I shall label them, 'absolute' properties. Let us call this *the casuistical resource*. It bases action and policy on such a concept's applying or failing to apply, and while there is room for border-line cases of various kinds there will be no way in which the concept can apply to a greater or lesser degree. (*Being dead* is an example of an absolute property: there may be borderline cases, but one cannot say that one person is more—or less—dead than another.) On this schema, the appearance of a slippery-slope argument will have a significance going beyond any that I have explained. It will show that distinctions are not being based on the right kinds of consideration at all.

This set of ideas deserves closer scrutiny than I can provide here, but 'absolute' properties are notoriously of different kinds, and even brief reflection suggests that merely by being absolute they cannot solve these problems of ethical decision. Thus it is true (to take once more the example that so often appears in these discussions) that one thing cannot be more of a human being than another, but there are at least two different possibilities that may underlie that truth. The more radical is that a thing which is at any time a human being has always been a human being, and nothing can turn into a human being from being something else. The less radical is that something can indeed become a human being, but that the stages that it goes through in the course of doing that do not involve being less or more of a human being.

If we base a concept of 'human being' on the second, less radical, construction, and this is then embodied in a rule about (for instance) abortion, we shall not avoid the problems of the slippery slope. All that we shall have done is to make the resolution of those problems by fixing a time seem all the more arbitrary. The rationale of the rule will be that one should not kill a human being, while the content of the rule is that one should not perform an abortion after a certain time. But no one can claim that a foetus becomes a human being at (just) that time, so if there is great insistence on the absolute character of the property that gives the rule its rationale, it will seem arbitrary that the rule should have that content.

What this approach does is to sharpen the normative predicate; refuse—reasonably—to sharpen the concept of 'human being'; and insist at the same time that the normative predicate must be directly and exclusively governed by that concept, as opposed to drawing the line there because a line is needed and that is no worse place to draw it than any other. To avoid this conflict, those who make the last of those requirements may insist that the concept of 'human being' should be based on the first and more radical construction, which has the result that any fertilized ovum is a human being, and (effectively) no abortion is allowed. It may be that the reason for adopting this concept and applying it in this way can be found from independent sources. Certainly they will need to carry great authority if we are to accept in such an important question this interpretation of the concept (and, by implication, of other notions that involve growth and development) when we would not find such an interpretation at all natural or convincing in other connections. But an entirely independent argument is rarely heard. Some appeal is usually made to the slippery-slope consequences of using the less radical interpretation. But once the problem is honestly faced in these terms, the casuistical resource seems a great deal less compelling, and it is better to consider directly whether there is a slippery slope, and, if so, how to deal with it.

There are some absolute terms, the absolute character of which is really only a verbal matter, a substantival wrap for a content which is basically comparative. 'A wit', 'a giant', and (unless it refers to a profession) 'a cricketer' are examples, and there are many more, reflection on which will show how little help we get with slippery-slope arguments merely by appealing to absolute rather than to frankly comparative notions. A very important and misleading example is 'person', as that term is sometimes used by philosophers in ethical connections.[5] It is formally true that no one can be more of a person than anyone else, but almost all the characteristics associated by those philosophers with being a person, such as the capacities for responsible action, for relations with others, for first-personal reflection, and so on, come in degrees. Moreover, they come in different degrees, and are not simply correlated with each other, nor with different ages, states of mental health, or other such attributes.

This concept, despite its absolute appearance, will provide no firm basis for rules about killing and similar matters, and those who place faith in it are deceiving themselves. What degree of what characteristic will count in a given context for being a person may very well turn out to be a function of the interests involved—other people's interests, in many cases. Certainly there is no slippery slope more perilous than that extended by a concept which is falsely supposed not to be slippery.

7 THE ARTIFICIAL FAMILY[1]

MARY WARNOCK

At the outset, there are two preliminary remarks I should like to make. First, I am not altogether satisfied with the title of this lecture. The notion of an artificial family may suggest something that is man-made, contrived, and somehow necessarily inferior to the supposed natural product with which it is contrasted (rather as, in my childhood, there was a material called 'artificial silk', words uttered in tones of scorn and snobbish derision by those of my mother's generation, and quite properly, since it was horrible and very inferior stuff). I am, however, in want of a better term to describe families which differ from the accepted norm of the family, as depicted in the cornflakes advertisements. Such families consist of mother, father, and children who are genetically related to both parents, and who were conceived in the usual way, by sexual intercourse. There are a number of ways in which the cornflakes family may in fact differ from this norm without being particularly unusual, still less abnormal. For example the children may be genetically related to the mother but not to the mother's husband, for they may be the children of a previous marriage and he the stepfather, or they may have been the children of an adulterous relationship. Or the children may be socially the children of both parents but genetically related to neither, having been adopted. These kinds of family come under my general heading 'artificial', though I shall not be saying anything more about them. I mention them only to put the kinds of family I am going to talk about in a proper, wider context. Secondly, the problems I am going to discuss are problems of medical ethics, but in what is perhaps a rather odd way. They do not arise precisely out of a doctor's duty to treat the sick. In some ways they should be seen as social problems which happen sometimes (though not always or not necessarily) to involve the medical profession, and on which doctors must therefore make up their minds like the rest of us. Part of the question I want to raise, however, is this: how much special power should the medical profession have, within society as a whole, and within the framework of the law? The sense of this question will, I hope, become clear as I consider three different forms of 'artificial' or non-normal ways of starting a family.

First, then, the family may be established by means of *in vitro* fertilization. The original test-tube baby, the first to be born anywhere in the world, was Louise Brown, born in Oldham in 1978, as a result of years of attempts by Patrick Steptoe and Robert Edwards. Since 1978 a substantial number of other babies have been born by this means all over the world. The theory of *in vitro* fertilization is simple, the practice very tricky. A ripe egg is extracted by surgical operation from a woman's ovary just before it would have been released by nature. It is mixed with the semen of the husband in a dish and fertilization occurs. The fertilized egg is then transferred back to the uterus, once it has started to divide. The recovery of the egg, its culture outside the body, the retransfer of the developing embryo to the uterus are all difficult. The timing, the temperature, the exact nature of the medium within which fertilization will take place, the right moment for the reintroduction of the embryo into the womb, all need to be very precisely controlled. Although it is claimed that of the hundreds of operations that have been carried out at Bourne Hall, where Steptoe and Edwards now work, there is a 25 per cent success rate, it is by no means certain that all these pregnancies have resulted in live births. Nor is it clear how many women have been operated on more than once. Though for women with severely damaged fallopian tubes, or none, *in vitro* fertilization may represent the only hope at present of their becoming pregnant, it is a long and stressful business which may very well lead to disappointment in the end. It is to be hoped, however, that as time goes on techniques will improve and success rates with them.

As is well known, the birth of Louise Brown caused great excitement, and rightly so. People were amazed at the immense patience and skill which had gone into the process, but also at the possibilities which they saw opening up for science and research: uneasiness was as widespread as admiration. Part of the uneasiness arose from the fact that it became suddenly clear that there would exist in the laboratory a number of 'spare' embryos, which might or might not be introduced into the uterus. These embryos would have come into existence through the use of drugs to produce 'superovulation', in which several eggs are produced by a woman in the same cycle, and can be collected at the same time, by means of a single surgical operation. All the eggs can then be fertilized, but only some introduced into the uterus. The rest can then be frozen and may be used for research, or introduced into the uterus either of the original woman or another, at a later date.

I don't want to embark on any kind of slippery-slope argument, which in any case has already been considered in Chapter 6. I would just say that it was the use of spare embryos that seemed to many to be the beginning of the slope, and public fears still centre on this problem. From the point of view of the family, it is relevant to say that in theory it would now be possible for a wife to give birth to her husband's child years after he was dead. Only four successful pregnancies have so far resulted from frozen embryos;[2] the freezing of embryos has, however, become almost routine in the breeding of livestock, and it is surely only a matter of time before the same techniques become common practice among human beings. In any case, the same result is possible if the husband's sperm is frozen before his death.[3] In theory, too, it is possible that an embryo, fertilized *in vitro* in 1985, could be introduced into a woman's womb, and born in 2085. The result would emphatically be a non-cornflakes family. It strikes me personally as a curious rather than a horrifying possibility. But others may think differently.[4]

If the techniques of IVF are improved and are more certain of success it may become possible to use them for the purposes of a new-style family planning. For instance, an embryo fertilized *in vitro* may be divided when it contains two or four cells. Each cell will then of course develop into a separate individual or clone with identical characteristics and genetic composition to that of its siblings derived from the same embryo. Cloning could be used to investigate the chromosomal normality of human embryos conceived by a couple who have a high chance of procreating an abnormal child. All the clones except one would be frozen; one would then be allowed to develop until it was possible to determine whether the embryo had the normal chromosomal complement, or, for example, the extra chromosome that is diagnostic of Down's syndrome. If the embryo was found to be abnormal, the frozen clones would not be transferred; if it was found to be normal, one or more could be unfrozen and transferred to the mother's uterus. (Unless ethical considerations were thought to dictate otherwise, the embryo used for the test would then presumably be discarded, or else used for research, since it would have passed the optimum stage of development for being transferred to the womb.) It has been suggested, too, that IVF, cloning, and freezing could be used to determine the sex of an embryo, before its transfer to the mother's uterus, where there is a risk of an inherited sex-linked disorder such as haemophilia. Again, it is on the horizon that, in the future, without cloning, an embryo fertilized *in vitro* could be examined for a single defective gene, for example that which gives rise to cystic fibrosis;[5] if discovered, this gene might ultimately be replaced by a normal gene. And so on. On we go down the slope. Such possibilities would give rise to families in some sense 'artificial'. They would certainly, by means of medical intervention, greatly reduce the number of severely handicapped families. And my personal view is that such an outcome is greatly to be desired.

Let us, however, return from the brink. Let us consider what is possible now: the IVF family. The first thing to be noticed here is that for such a family to exist a great deal of medical skill and expertise has to be deployed; and the parents of the family have to be stoical, level-headed, optimistic, and yet prepared for failure. They also have to have plenty of time (or at least the mother has). But if all these conditions are satisfied, it is hard to see any problems specific to successful cases of IVF. The child is born after a pregnancy like any other, once implantation has taken place, and he is genetically the offspring of both his parents. The fact that surgical intervention has to take place to get the pregnancy started may come to seem no more remarkable than that sometimes, at the other end of pregnancy, there has to be surgery in order that the baby can be born. If we look at IVF itself, then, as a remedy for certain kinds of infertility, and apart from any spin-off, there seem to be no objections to it, and no ethical questions to be raised.[6] There may, however, be problems related to provision; to these I shall return.

The second kind of family I want to consider is that formed by means of artificial insemination. In certain rare cases the donor of semen may be the husband of the woman who is to be inseminated (AIH). But usually, when we think of artificial insemination, we think of a donor who is other than the husband (AID); and obviously the primary use for artificial insemination is where the husband himself is infertile. It is difficult to say with any precision how common AID is, but a fair guess would be that about a thousand children are born of such pregnancies every year in this country. But the number may be higher; for the crucial fact about AID is that it is an easy method to use. All that is needed is a man willing to produce semen by masturbation, and a syringe by means of which it can be introduced into the vagina close to the cervix, near the time of ovulation. It is simple and highly likely to succeed, even at the first attempt.

I emphasize the simplicity, because it will be seen that there need be no medical intervention in the whole process. Do-it-yourself kits are on sale. The woman who becomes pregnant by this means will then of course seek medical attention in the ordinary way, but her doctor need never know how she became pregnant. Nevertheless, at present one must assume that most AID families are the result of insemination in a medical context, with sperm donated anonymously, probably frozen, and used by a doctor for insemination. The doctor will have had the task of advising the woman about AID and seeing to it that the facilities are available.

Though AID was a known process for humans as much as a hundred years ago (for other animals it has been used for much longer), it became a subject of open debate only in the 1950s, when various committees were set up to discuss it. The Feversham Committee, which reported in 1960,[7] was highly critical of the practice, and plainly wished that it did not exist, but recognized that it could not be prohibited by law. They contented themselves with recommending that it be discouraged. In 1981 a book called *The Artificial Family* came out, by Dr Snowden and Professor Mitchell from the Institute of Population Studies at Exeter, who again examined the problems of AID and (for the reasons set out below) were pessimistic in their findings, with regard to the family.[8] This has been followed by a second book, *Artificial Reproduction*, by the same authors, in which they come to essentially the same conclusions as previously.[9] The arguments against AID are, first, that it produces an asymmetry in the family relations. The children are the genetic offspring of the mother, but not of the father, and a third figure (albeit a shadowy and anonymous figure) has been introduced into what ought to be the two-person relation of marriage. If the marriage breaks up after the birth of the children, the husband may feel no responsibility for the children who are, according to the present law, illegitimate. (There is, however, no doubt that the law will, in this respect, be changed.[10]) The motivation of the donor was also questioned by the Feversham Committee. But the main argument that Snowden and Mitchell use against AID is the secrecy with which it takes place, and the deception generally involved, starting with the common falsification of the birth certificate[11] and continuing, as often as not, with the pretence both to the child himself and to the immediate family that the child is the genetic offspring of both parents. Moreover, doctors themselves tend to be caught up in this web of deception, and sometimes appear to argue that medical confidentiality enjoins them to conceal the husband's infertility. It can be seen that the problems surrounding the AID family are social rather than strictly medical, yet doctors may frequently be involved in making decisions, in particular about who is to receive treatment, and how they are to be advised.

Before discussing these considerations further, I will briefly describe a third form of artificial family, of which there are probably few examples, namely the family formed by the use of a surrogate mother. I will not weary you with all the various different genetic combinations and methods of impregnation possible in the case of surrogacy. But two obvious kinds of family might be where a sperm and egg are fertilized *in vitro*, and the embryo is implanted in a woman who will provide an environment within which the embryo can develop normally, will give birth to a child to which she has made no genetic contribution, and will hand over the child at birth to its genetic parents. Alternatively, a man may contribute sperm with which a woman (who is not his wife) is inseminated. The child born is thus genetically the husband's but not the wife's. It is partly the child of the woman who bears it. This kind of surrogacy has been described as the flip side of AID. There is probably a considerable number of couples for whom this kind of family is the only chance they have of a child even half genetically their own. All the objections raised against the AID family have been urged against the surrogacy family, and more besides. For it is argued that the intrusion of a third person into the marriage relation is far more damaging where that person is a woman who goes through nine months of pregnancy in making her contribution. The donor of sperm, in contrast, is totally impersonal as well as anonymous. Moreover there is a very strong feeling that a woman who acts as a surrogate is being, if not exploited (for she will have chosen so to act and will certainly be paid) at least used as a means to someone else's end, and that this is intrinsically immoral. This feeling is far stronger where it is a woman who becomes pregnant on someone else's behalf than where it is a case of a man giving sperm, a quick and probably easily forgettable experience, not entailing the great physical changes and deep psychological involvement associated with pregnancy. And apart from abstract questions of morality, there are numerous practical difficulties about surrogacy which do not arise in the case of AID. The mother who carries the child and gives birth to it may for example change her mind, and want to keep it despite her contract.[12] The child may, on the other hand, because it is born handicapped or because of a change in circumstances, in the end be wanted by neither party. The law is not at present clear how to proceed in cases of dispute but it is unlikely to uphold any surrogacy contract in court.[13]

Once again we have a whole series of problems, none of them (except the original infertility problem) strictly medical, but with which, at some stage or other, a doctor may have to tangle. It is time to turn, then, to the doctor's proper role. It seems to me that there are two types of problem, in this field, with which doctors are likely to become involved. First, there is a question, often raised, which they are obliged to answer: 'Do patients who are infertile merit treatment?' Now this is a question which is of interest partly because there is an intrinsic difference between the way doctors are likely to answer it and the way that at least somewhat theoretically inclined members of the public will answer it. If a patient, or a couple of patients, come to their doctor and say that they have failed to conceive a child and want to do so, then no doctor is likely to turn them away as not deserving of treatment.

On the other hand, there is a fair number of lay people who will say that there are too many children in the world anyway, and that infertility is a minor affliction for which, on the whole, we should be thankful. In any case, no one ever died of infertility, so it cannot be an urgent case for treatment even if it deserves treatment at all. I have heard such views very seriously canvassed.[14] They cannot be disregarded. If, however, we assume that most doctors, because of their commitment to their individual patients, whose needs come above any global considerations, will say 'yes' to treating infertility, the question still remains by what means they should treat it, or how far they should go: are they to draw a line in treatment beyond which they will not proceed? Such questions must to some extent be matters of finance. In this respect there is no difference between how far to go in treating infertility, and how far to go, let us say, in operating on people with crooked noses, or even keeping people alive on life-support machines. It is all, as the cliché phrase has it, a matter of priorities.

It is my belief that the question of how much money to allocate for this or that branch of medicine must be settled at a district or perhaps regional level. In practice, the answer will not be theoretical but contingent, or accidental. A regional hospital board will spend more on aspects of medicine in which they know that they have expertise. They will, moreover, be bullied into expending more resources by those doctors who have powerful personalities and enthusiasm, and can show prestigious evidence of their success in a particular field. I do not believe that such accidents of fortune can be eliminated from the issue of how much money should be spent on this or that. But because of the wholly contingent nature of questions of priority, I do not propose to discuss them further. (And I think my committee was right to refuse to consider any question the answer to which was to be that a particular percentage of resources should be allocated to this or that or the other treatment.)

But sometimes the question 'How far shall I go?' must be a different kind of question. Suppose there is a doctor whose patient, a woman, is congenitally malformed, in that she has no uterus. She is married, let us say, and she and her husband are desperate. She knows that she can never bear a child, but she wants, for both their sakes, to have his child. The doctor she consults knows that the only possibility for them is to use a surrogate to bear her husband's child. What does he do? We can imagine various alternative hypotheses. He, the doctor, disapproves wholly of surrogacy. He regards it as a form of exploitation analogous to prostitution. Knowing that such an arrangement would be possible, he nevertheless does not discuss it with his patient. For to do so would be to encourage something he believes to be absolutely wrong. (I have heard a medical student, in a similar way, say that he would refuse to cause superovulation in a patient of his even though such superovulation would make it possible to increase her chances of a successful IVF pregnancy. For he thought that every embryo fertilized should be implanted in the uterus, none should be spare; therefore not only would he not be a party to the production of spare embryos, but he would not tell his patient that other doctors might feel differently.) Again, there might by now, in our imagined case, be a change in the law, such that to advertise a surrogacy service was a criminal offence.[15] Our doctor, however, believes that he must offer his patient a chance of a child if that is what she deeply wants, so he says 'I can probably find you a surrogate, among my students, who would carry a child for you.' He is not, under the supposed law, committing a criminal offence, nor will the couple who contract with the girl be committing any offence. And he thinks it is his duty to offer this chance to his patient. If they can fix up a contract, good luck to them. Is he right? From the standpoint of medical ethics, where a doctor's first duty is to his patient, I believe he is.

The problem here is that the medical profession has a tendency to regard 'medical ethics' in a narrowly professional light. And they are not to be blamed for this. They start from some limiting premiss, such as the so-called Hippocratic Oath (which of course is a potent form of myth, differently interpreted by different doctors; even if such an oath had a clear historical existence over the centuries, why should it still be binding, unless people wanted to be bound by some such mythological chains?) and from this premiss they deduce a certain duty to their patients, but no particular duty to society at large. If anything, it is a matter of doctor and patient *contra mundum*. Doctors often express this kind of sentiment by saying that though of course they are interested in acting ethically, they are not interested in morals. (Or if they are interested, for themselves, it is not part of their business to discuss morals with their patients, still less to impose morality on them.) It is, however, less than clear to me what this alleged distinction between ethics and morals is supposed to be. Let us assume that medical ethics is a wholly professional concept concerned with the agreed right treatment of a patient, or at least with a kind of presumed integrity of purely professional judgement. Then 'morals' will comprehend everything else considered right or wrong. It will comprehend all that a doctor thinks is good or bad in non-professional, non-therapeutic contexts. Very well then: a doctor, like the rest of us, must have some ideas, however vague, about the kind of society he thinks good. Are these ideas to have no bearing at all on his practice? Suppose he believes, for example, that our supposed law with regard to surrogacy is too restrictive of freedom.[16] Should he act, or advise his patients to act, in contravention of the law? Or, if his moral view is stricter than the law, should he refuse to treat his patients in what is a legitimate way, on the ground that the law is too liberal?

There is an equally important and related question which may face the medical practitioner. It is the question of the scope of provision of artificial families. First, a doctor may think it his duty to ensure that fertility services are provided only for those who are fit to become parents. For, he may argue, a couple who wish to adopt a child are put through any number of tests, they submit to innumerable interviews and all kinds of most personal scrutiny before they are deemed fit. Why should those who want their child in a different way be less carefully scrutinized? Yet such scrutiny seems intolerably intrusive. Do we want doctors to carry it out? Do we really want it carried out at all? That couples may, to a greater degree than ever before, choose to become parents does not entail that they should undergo tests of fitness which, in the old days when such things lay in the lap of the gods, they did not have to undergo. Which of us who had our children in the ordinary way would have survived such scrutiny, if we had been obliged to submit to it? There is much talk about 'counsel-ling' for those couples who wish, or think they wish, to embark on IVF, AID, or surrogacy. And it is certainly necessary that no couple should embark on such things without fully understanding what they are up to, and what is their chance of success. But beyond this, I personally doubt whether 'counselling' has a place. For all the claim that counselling is essentially value-free, I doubt whether it can occur without some message being picked up, perhaps mistakenly, by the subject of counselling, that one course of action ought to be preferred to another. I have heard a doctor claim that he always counsels those who come to him for a cure for infertility; and he often counsels them until they go away. Certainly, if doctors have to decide which couples to treat, which not, they are embarking on a course which is miles away from 'medical ethics', but essentially discriminatory, and discriminatory on social or moral grounds.

That this is so becomes even clearer if we consider a second case—that of the doctor requested to provide services, AID say, for someone who is not part of the ordinary cornflakes family at all, and never likely to be: the homosexual, for example, or the single woman, or the lesbian couple, any of whom may, increasingly, come to demand a child as of right, a child to be born by surrogacy or AID. Such persons are in no way sick. They are not infertile, as far as the doctor may know. They simply want the service available to the infertile to be available to them. They regard it as a right, either to father a child whom they can bring up, or to bear a child whom they can bring up. Is the doctor to provide the service?

It seems to me that matters would in some ways be easier for the doctor if all services of the kind in question were available at certain agreed, licensed centres.[17] For, if this were so, at least no doctor in general practice would be obliged to establish his own criteria for accepting or rejecting people for the service. He could simply point everyone in the direction of the local centre. This is of course to pass the buck only a very little way down. On the other hand, it might be easier to establish uniform practice at a small number of regional centres than among countless numbers of individual GPs; and those seeking the services would have less reason to feel aggrieved if they ended up not getting what they wanted if they had sought the service at a recognized and legitimized centre. They could not so easily blame personal prejudice.

There would be other obvious advantages. If centres were established regionally, subject to the granting of a licence, users would be assured that the sperm stored there came from properly screened donors; also that there would be a check on how many times a particular donor's sperm was used, and that advice would be available if it was needed. Such centres might also keep a list of the names of possible surrogate mothers. It could gradually become established that, though anonymity of donors remains highly desirable, secrecy and deception are not. Just as adopted children are these days nearly always told that they are adopted, so parents could be urged to tell the truth to their AID or surrogate-born children. Obviously, no law can enforce such openness. But the climate of opinion at a well-run centre could be very influential.

Some of the burdens would thereby be lifted from individual medical practitioners. They would have one set of conflicts the fewer, between their duty to an individual patient, and what they may think of as a duty to society as a whole. For there is no doubt that the centre of anxiety for most people, and therefore presumably for many doctors, is whether we actually like the idea of a society within which all these different kinds of families are acceptable. Some people (Dr Snowden and Professor Mitchell among these) doubt whether being born into such a family is in the best interests of the child. Other people have more vague and diffuse doubts about the possible effects on the institution of the family as such. For they think of the family as mother, father, and children, all genetically bound to one another, as well as to aunts, uncles, and grandparents. They are aware that there are many other patterns of family life, as we saw at the beginning, but they still regard the traditional pattern as ideal.

There is no doubt that the word 'family' is a highly emotive word. In some contexts, including run-of-the-mill political contexts, it is enough simply to use the word, however vaguely. It is like 'democracy' or 'freedom'. We all have to be for it. Recently, however, there have been assaults on the family, from psychiatrists and, above all these days, from feminists, who regard it as the source of all tension, a bastion of male domination, a way of defining a role for women and keeping them within it. To be able to have children in some other context, to open the doors and windows on the tightly bound little group, has become, for some people, an ideal in itself. The new possibilities offered by AID and surrogacy are there to be explored in the cause of social reform. They should not be regarded solely as a less-than-perfect solution to the problems of the infertile.

Often those who attempt to defend the concept of the family against such assaults have little to say in its defence except that it has always existed as the source and origin of human affection, the seed-bed of human sympathy, without which morality itself could not come into being. Whether that is necessarily true, whether things could be otherwise, has not, in the nature of the case, been fully explored.

Certain fairly well-established facts may be thought relevant here. It seems to be generally agreed that a child is better off in a family than in care, that he needs above everything a person to whom he can become attached and of whose affection for himself he feels assured. It is equally widely accepted that it does not very much matter who this person is.[18] Foster-parents, for example, or adoptive parents, provide an environment generally far better than an ill-named 'home', however good. They may often do better, too, than parents genetically related to the child. Such considerations might make one argue that, provided children are brought up by a grown-up who wants them and shows affection, it does not really matter within what kind of group they live: cosiness is all.

Beliefs concerning the importance of a child's having male and female models are less easy to evaluate, though no less frequently expressed. It might be that further research could throw light on this, and on the question whether or not it is important for a child to have siblings. To be the only child either with one adult or with a group may seem less than ideal for a child. But there is not very much evidence here to back up intuitions.

All such considerations, all talk of 'evidence', suggests that there is a relatively clear way of assessing the well-being or interests of the child. The anxieties expressed, for example, by Snowden and Mitchell might thus be allayed if it could be shown that children actually benefit, or may do so, from the new kinds of family. The criterion would be broadly utilitarian, with perhaps extra weight given to the happiness of the child compared with that of the parents, since the child, if unhappy, could be seen as the innocent victim of someone else's whim. That, of course, is a non-utilitarian reason for attaching additional weight to the happiness of the child—a reason appealing to considerations of justice. But it seems to me that there are, in fact, good utilitarian reasons for thinking that, as a matter of practical policy, the misery of a miserable child should count for more than the satisfaction of one, or perhaps even two, grown-ups. I have in mind, first, the wealth of evidence suggesting that unhappiness in childhood is likely to stand in the way of proper emotional adjustment in later life; and secondly, the likely consequences for society of allowing numbers of children to be brought up miserably. Misery, it is said, breeds misery; but, in general, this is truer, I should have thought, of misery in children than it is of misery in adults. (The adoption of a policy of differential weighting need not be regarded, therefore, as inconsistent with maintaining, at the theoretical level, Bentham's dictum 'everybody to count for one, nobody for more than one'.)

Nevertheless, in considering not individual families, and their share of happiness or the reverse, but the family in general, and its place within society, it seems much less easy to find utilitarian backing for either pessimism or optimism in the face of possible change. One thing is certain: considering ourselves as a whole society, we shall in future have far more choices open to us than ever before, in the range of possible family life. And being able to choose things necessarily brings moral problems, where perhaps there were none before. Our attitude to disaster, or even to mere discomfort or discontent, is different if we feel that it could have been avoided. Thus in the old days infertility itself, though usually hard to become reconciled to, could have been regarded as a natural misfortune; and people who wanted children, but could not have them, adapted themselves by adopting or by otherwise making the best of things. Increasingly, if it is seen that infertility can be remedied, it will equally be felt that to do nothing is blameworthy. Previously, if people chose to live as homosexuals, they thereby chose not to have children, something they perhaps regretted, but which was a part of the larger choice. Now, if surrogacy becomes a genuine option, there is a further choice to make, whether to have a family by means of a surrogate. Then again, the birth of a handicapped child used to be an unforeseeable disaster (and to a large extent still is so). But perhaps with the improvement of the techniques involved in *in vitro* fertilization, and consequential processes, it will be possible to ensure that the embryo is non-defective before transferring it to the mother's womb. Such techniques already, of course, make it theoretically possible for parents to choose the sex of their children.[19] And so on. Already, in America, commercial sperm banks are offering women the choice of having children who are genetically the children of the kind of men they admire: athletes, Nobel prize winners, violinists.[20] There are two separate difficulties about making such choices. First, how to weigh up the advantages and disadvantages in each particular case; but secondly, how to compare short-term satisfaction with possible long-term consequences for society. When we are faced with such massively difficult calculations, where the unknown factors are literally innumerable, the principle of utility (the principle that we should so act as to maximize benefit and minimize harm) offers little or no practical guidance. Does it follow, then, that where public policy, policy for a whole society, is in question, utilitarianism should be abandoned? Should we instead seek a kind of consensus, derived from what people vaguely feel about their origins, their roots, their commitments to their own children, however awkward and unsatisfactory their non-Nobel-prize-winning genes may turn out to be? Are we simply to try to think what sort of society we would feel it tolerable or intolerable to live in?

I suspect that in the end this is what we must do. But then, of course, the question is: Who are 'we' supposed to be? Boringly, I suppose that the answer is that we are the people who elect MPs, and who indeed *are* MPs, and magistrates, parliamentary draftsmen, Judges, Lords of Appeal, and all the various persons concerned in the making of law and its enforcement.

So where, among all this varied lot, does the medical profession fit in? It seems to me that doctors have a double problem. First, they have to reconcile what they conceive to be the good of their patients with the good of society. This, of course, is not a new problem for them, nor one which is uniquely connected with the artificial family. It occurs just as often, for example, in connection with the treatment of mental illness (should a patient be treated against his will?). The factor which may make it especially hard for a doctor to answer that question in the present case is that he must not think just of his patient on one side and society on the other but uneasily, in between, of the unborn child.

Secondly, doctors have to consider what is for the good of society? What sort of society do they want to see? Now as far as this second problem goes we are all, as I hope to have suggested, in the same boat. I do not believe that doctors have any special role to play in determining, or even in influencing, public policy. We are all entitled to our bit of influence, or even of decision-making. I hold, of course, that doctors are as much entitled to their opinions as the rest of us when it comes to the sanctity or otherwise of the traditional family. But I do not believe that their moral feelings, however sincere and deeply felt, should be allowed any special weight in such matters. Nor do I believe that most doctors want to be forced into decision-making which is outside their professional sphere.

It is precisely for this reason that I think, on grounds of political theory, that the provision of services which will result in the artificial family should be made in licensed centres and only there. For then the terms on which the licences will be granted, the inspection of the centres, and the changing of the conditions of licence from time to time will all be ultimately the responsibility of the Minister in whose province such things fall. And the legislation that gives him such powers will have stemmed, not from medical opinion alone, but from Parliament. There is no other authority that we have any business to recognize.

Postscript on surrogate motherhood

In the discussion that followed this talk, I was pressed on the question of where precisely I stood on the much vexed question of surrogate motherhood. Let me repeat here the gist of what I said then. In some ways I am perhaps the wrong person to put this question to, since I personally hated being pregnant; and it was only getting a child at the end of the process that made it at all tolerable. I find it difficult to imagine a woman actually wanting to be pregnant in the knowledge and expectation of giving the child up to someone else, and I confess to finding it distinctly unappealing. But there is a larger issue that surrogacy raises.

One thing that being on the Committee of Inquiry has impressed upon me is the very widespread and deeply felt antipathy that there appears to be amongst the public at large towards the practice of surrogate motherhood. This emerged in one piece of evidence after another. Now I believe that morality cannot be separated from feelings. If people feel very deeply that they do not wish to live in the kind of society in which women regularly become pregnant for money, with the intention of giving the child away, then I believe that feeling deserves to be respected. In a democracy, I think people have a right to expect that it will be respected.

All this, of course, is a bit reminiscent of things that Lord Justice Devlin said, years ago, regarding homosexual practices between consenting adults,[21] in the wake of another Government Inquiry—that chaired by John Wolfenden.[22] Most philosophers at the time took a rather dim view of his arguments. But I'm not sure that homosexual practices and surrogacy are strictly parallel cases. For one thing, the opinion, such as it was, in favour of ensuring that homosexual practices between consenting adults should remain a crime, was very largely uneducated opinion. And for another, homosexual practices involve no third party, whereas surrogacy does, namely the child. His (or her) welfare is, from any point of view, something that the law may legitimately take into account. The legal difficulties, to look no further, that may arise from surrogacy have become more apparent, even since the report of my committee was published. I do not believe that any society should encourage the birth of children that, from the moment of birth, may be the subject of a bitter legal dispute.

But in any case, I disagree entirely with those philosophers who would claim, as did Professor Dworkin in response to Devlin's original article,[23] that feelings alone cannot amount to a moral view, and that morality has to be a matter of reason. (No doubt I am oversimplifying his position.) Indeed the whole notion of reason, on the one hand, and feeling or sentiment, on the other, essentially opposed to each other, seems to me to be a mistake—a hangover from an eighteenth-century way of looking at things. I don't see why a moral view cannot both be grounded in feelings and at the same time (in some suitably broad sense) be rational, or at any rate not irrational.

8 THE WARNOCK REPORT: A PHILOSOPHICAL APPRAISAL[1]

MICHAEL LOCKWOOD

The prospect of a philosopher chairing a government inquiry is one that fellow members of the profession are apt to view with somewhat mixed feelings. On the one hand, it is gratifying to think that the powers that be recognize and value the philosopher's peculiar kind of expertise; it is gratifying also to think that, for once, philosophy might actually impinge on the real world, that Parliamentary legislation might be guided by philosophical considerations (assuming that the Inquiry's recommendations are accepted and passed into law). But, on the other hand, philosophers disagree with one another. So, no doubt, do the members of all professions; but philosophers are apt to disagree at a rather more fundamental level than do physicists, say, or members of the medical profession. A fellow philosopher may well wonder, therefore, whether the philosophically trained chairman of a government committee is providing the right sort of philosophical guidance. Better no philosophy at all, he may even feel, than wrongheaded philosophy. This anxiety may be compounded by the consideration that the philosopher chairing the committee is very likely to be the only philosophically trained person there; things he or she might say, the contentiousness of which would be immediately apparent to a fellow member of the profession, are thus likely to go unchallenged. No doubt such thoughts are partly born of envy. Almost every philosopher, I suspect, would himself love to have been in Mary Warnock's position and by the same token is inwardly convinced that he himself would have done a simply splendid job; the Platonic conception of a philosopher king dies hard.

In a recent interview,[2] Mary Warnock was asked whether she had sometimes found herself, in effect, giving philosophy tutorials to other members of her Committee. She replied that she had, very frequently. So much so, she said (rather charmingly), that it got to the point at which, whenever philosophy was mentioned, people began to groan, rather like the lower fourth at the mention of Latin prose. (Not for nothing, it seems, was Mary Warnock once a headmistress.) In retrospect, she wondered whether she hadn't been 'a bit bossy'. What, one wonders, was she telling them? Was she gently chiding them for trying to derive an 'ought' from an 'is'? Was she busy detecting in their arguments fallacies of equivocation and the like? Or was some more substantive philosophical message put across? Certainly, the published report embodies a distinctive philosophical point of view. And one cannot doubt that it is largely Mary Warnock's own, seeing that it is a point of view that she has defended in several articles and interviews. It is that view that I am concerned to explore in this article. The view is, by her own account, partly a product of her time on the Inquiry rather than one that she simply brought to it.

The bulk of the recommendations in the Warnock Report seem to me both eminently sensible and also to have relatively little of interest to be said about them, from a philosophical standpoint. I shall therefore concentrate, in this article, on the two issues which are at once most controversial and in which questions of a recognizably philosophical character are most in evidence. I have in mind the issues of research on human embryos and of surrogate motherhood.

Embryo research

Many would suppose that the key question, when one is considering the ethics of scientific research using live human embryos, is 'Is the embryo a human being?' or perhaps 'Is it a person?'— 'When does human (or personal) life begin?' The thought, here, is that we have reasonably clear and agreed-upon views about what is and is not morally permissible, in the way of research, when dealing with individuals that are indisputably human beings or persons. Many of the things, perhaps all, that scientists are interested in doing to human embryos, for research purposes, would be universally regarded as unacceptable, if done to a child, say, or indeed to any other innocent human being without his or her consent. So if we knew at what stage the embryo becomes a human being or person, we should know that beyond that point, at any rate, the proposed research was morally impermissible.

The parallel might be challenged, of course, even by someone who was convinced that to experiment on a human embryo, at any stage in its development, is indeed to experiment on a human being. The early embryo, unlike a child, cannot suffer; and if it is not in any case going to be transferred to a womb, one might claim that it does not stand to lose by any physical injury done to it in the course of research. Nevertheless, it could be argued that if one really is dealing with a human being then experimenting on the human embryo constitutes a blatant violation of the Kantian principle that one should never treat a human being merely as a means to an end, but always as an end in itself: in short, it might be thought to be a morally unacceptable form of exploitation.

A further point is this. The death of an innocent human being is, other things being equal, something to be avoided. Thus it must be wrong, prima facie, to allow an embryo to develop beyond the point at which a human life begins, in circumstances in which that life is bound then to be prematurely extinguished. In keeping a human embryo alive in the laboratory beyond a certain point—whether for the purposes of experimentation or merely of observation is immaterial—the scientist would be doing just that. This may prompt the ingenious retort that almost anyone who has a child is indirectly bringing about the death of an innocent human being—since the child will, after all, one day die. But of course the point here is that the child's eventual death, regrettable though it is (Tom Nagel has remarked that 'a bad end is in store for us all'[3]), may reasonably be expected to be more than compensated for by the worthwhile life that precedes it. This can hardly be said of the death of an embryo in the laboratory.

For both these reasons, then, the question when human life begins, when we are dealing with a human being or person, might seem to be crucial here. But is it? One philosophical lesson that Mary Warnock would appear to have impressed successfully upon her fellow Committee members—so much so that it is staunchly asserted, not only in the majority Report, but also in a minority Expression of Dissent—is this: Questions such as 'When does life begin?', 'When does a human being come into existence?', and 'When does the embryo or foetus become a person?' are not straightforwardly factual questions at all. Roman Catholics, for example, who, taking the orthodox Vatican line, insist that what begins at conception is 'the life not of a potential human being but of a human being with potential'[4] are not making a purely factual claim—something which can, say, be tested empirically. No, what they are saying already covertly embodies a moral judgement, to the effect that the human embryo and foetus ought to be accorded the same degree of moral respect as we would accord to mature members of the human species. And the same, *mutatis mutandis*, would go for any other assertion as to when human (or personal) life begins: such claims are morally loaded. Hence they cannot, without circularity, be appealed to in order to help settle the question of what is or is not morally acceptable conduct in relation to the human embryo. One is best advised simply to set aside such pseudo-factual questions, and get on with trying to answer directly the straightforwardly evaluative question of how human embryos should be treated.

Regarding the matter in this light, so the argument continues, there are several things that can plausibly be said. First, the human embryo is at least a potential human being (in a sense of 'potential' that neither entails nor excludes 'actual'). That in itself ought, morally, to count for something. On this basis, the Report recommends 'that the embryo of the human species should be afforded some protection in law'.[5] Moreover, the further developed the embryo is, the further along the path to being incontrovertibly a human being, the weightier this claim for moral protection becomes. If I understand it correctly, the Report sees the human embryo as, in moral terms, occupying an initial segment of a continuous spectrum that has beings that are undeniably human beings or persons at the other end; the degree of moral respect owed to the developing embryo and foetus is, roughly speaking, a direct function of its level of development. Even very early human embryos are thus not, according to this view, morally negligible. Granted that even the very early embryo, since it has the potential for human life, is deserving of some moral consideration, there are, of course, other considerations too. The advancement of human knowledge, both in terms of the benefits to humankind that can be expected to result from it, and perhaps also in terms of its intrinsic worth, is a consideration that likewise deserves to be given moral weight. In thinking about the ethics of research on human embryos, these two sorts of consideration therefore have to be weighed against each other.

Some people, while accepting that the framework just sketched is an appropriate one for thinking about the issue, may nevertheless feel that the moral protection deserved by the human embryo in virtue of its potential for human life outweighs considerations about advancing scientific knowledge right from the outset, so that research on live human embryos ought never to be permitted. That is precisely the view put forward in one Expression of Dissent.[6] Others—and this is the majority view expressed in the Report—will think that at a sufficiently early stage the balance of considerations is in favour of allowing some research to be carried out: serious research, that is, research that has the potential for making a substantial contribution to scientific knowledge. Inevitably, however, as we consider embryos at more and more advanced stages of development, the scales will at some point tip the other way: the protection of the embryo then comes to be the paramount consideration, and a point is reached beyond which research ought no longer to be permitted.

Putting things this way, of course, there is no reason to suppose that the point at which the scales tip will be the same for every piece of research that someone might have in mind; the greater the value of the research, the later in embryonic development it might be thought right to permit it to take place (always supposing that the research required embryos at that advanced a stage of development). Realistically, however, it would be neither practical nor satisfactory to try to decide these matters on a case-by-case basis. Nor, in matters such as this, where sensitivity to human life itself is at stake, can we leave it to the discretion of scientists or research-ethics committees, however well-intentioned they might be. The possibilities of abuse are too great. If understandable public anxiety on these matters is to be allayed, one must simply draw a rigid line somewhere and make sure that nobody is allowed to cross it. The Report is insistent on the need for 'barriers'.[7]

Precisely where the line is to be drawn, given that embryonic development is an essentially continuous process, is, the Report concedes, bound to be to some extent arbitrary, in the light of the above considerations. However, there is something to be said for choosing fourteen days as the cut-off point, seeing that this is just before the point of formation of the 'primitive streak' which later becomes the spinal cord. It is generally believed that division of the embryo, to produce identical twins, triplets, or whatever, is impossible beyond that point. Before then, as Mary Warnock put it in a recent interview, 'the embryo hasn't yet decided how many people it is going to be'. There is thus a sense in which we are not yet dealing with a fully determinate individual.

This I take to be the line of argument that issues in the following key proposals:

We accordingly recommend that no live human embryo derived from in vitro fertilisation, whether frozen or unfrozen, may be kept alive, if not transferred to a woman, beyond fourteen days after fertilisation, nor may it be used as a research subject beyond fourteen days after fertilisation. This fourteen day period does not include any time during which the embryo may have been frozen. We further recommend that it shall be a criminal offence to handle or to use as a research subject any live human embryo derived from in vitro fertilisation beyond that limit.[8]

I have done my best to present this line of thought in as sympathetic and persuasive a way as I can—making explicit, in the process, things which I take to be implicit in the Report itself. But I am bound to say that the argument seems to me to be philosophically flawed. In the first place, while it is perfectly true that terms such as 'life', 'person', and 'human being' are very often, in this context, used in a way that is morally question-begging, it is not clear to me that they have to be used in this way; or (which some would take to be the second horn of the philosophical dilemma here) that if they are not so used such terms then become simply irrelevant to deciding the moral issue. More of that in a moment.

I am, secondly, unconvinced that any moral significance should be attached to primitive-streak formation, even granted that this represents the last moment at which embryonic division can occur. To be sure, there is a venerable tradition, both in philosophy and theology, that human beings are, as a matter of logical necessity, indivisible. (This was argued, for example, by both Descartes and Leibniz.[9] Descartes, indeed, took this supposed indivisibility as a proof of mind–body dualism: since the body clearly is divisible, it followed, he thought, that he was distinct from his body.[10]) If the pre-fifteen-day embryo is divisible and persons are not, then it may seem to follow that, before fifteen days at any rate, there is no human being associated with the embryo.

Strictly, of course, this does not follow; embryonic division might be correlated with the coming into existence, in association with one of the two halves, of a new human being altogether. Or, if it is thought an objection to this that it introduces a gratuitous asymmetry into what is ostensibly a symmetrical process, perhaps the original human being is destroyed by the division and supplanted by two new ones. We may waive this point. (The question of how many souls are implicated in the division of an embryo is the sort of thing that would commend itself to someone who is becoming bored with the problem of how many angels can stand on the head of a pin.)

A far more serious objection to the argument is that its premiss seems likely to be false. For there is considerable evidence that human beings are divisible, not only as a matter of logical possibility (that it is logically impossible for human beings to divide was never a very plausible claim), but as a matter of fact. In saying this, I have in mind the celebrated 'split brain' experiments of Sperry and others,[11] in which strikingly dissociated behaviour has been evoked in patients with a severed corpus callosum, the bridge of tissue that normally joins the two hemispheres of the brain. In experimental situations in which it is contrived that different information passes into the two hemispheres, such patients behave in a way that has led Sperry himself and several other workers in the field to conclude that the two hemispheres of their brains are associated with distinct streams of consciousness. (Nor is such behaviour confined to such artificially devised situations: in one famous case, the patient's right hand would embrace his wife, while the left attempted to push her away!) Sperry's own interpretation of the evidence is, admittedly, not universally accepted; but it would seem perverse, in the face of these phenomena, to maintain that human beings are essentially indivisible.[12] Even if, as some have claimed, the behavioural dissociation in 'split-brain' patients is not quite total, it could almost certainly be made so by severing fibres lower down. So divisibility is, I suggest, a red herring here: if very early embryos are to be regarded as non-human beings by virtue of their divisibility, then so, probably, should I be.

That, in any case, is by the way. The heart of the issue lies in the questions whether the potentiality for human (or personal) life inherent in the human embryo really does, as the Warnock Report assumes, confer on it any moral standing and whether one really can, if one is to do justice to this issue, avoid confronting the question when human life begins. I believe that the answer to both questions is 'No'. I have argued this at length in Chapter 1 and am reluctant to repeat myself. Briefly, however, the key points seem to me to be these. First, talk of potentiality is crucially ambiguous in this context. A child may think of himself as a potential astronaut, star footballer, or (in an earlier generation) engine-driver. Here to be a potential X is potentially to be an X: the child, in the unlikely event of his actually becoming an astronaut, say, is the very same individual as that future astronaut.

If, at a given stage of embryonic development, we could say, in this sense, that we had a potential person—something that (assuming that it will develop into a being with the capacity for reflective self-consciousness, rational thought, and so forth) can be regarded as the very same individual as that future being—then it is clear why one should suppose that this conferred on it a certain moral standing. Given that the attributes that mark us off from other animals are ones which, on the whole, we think of ourselves as being very fortunate to possess, we can see that it is very much in the interests of a being with the potential to develop them and to enjoy the kind of life that they make possible, that this potentiality be allowed to come to fruition. Correspondingly, then, it is clear why one should think it wrong to kill a being with such potential, and by extension, wrong to bring into existence an individual with such potential in circumstances where the potential was not going to be realized. This, it could plausibly be argued, is the kind of interest that confers a moral claim—and thus an interest which should (other things being equal) both be respected, when we encounter it, and not be brought into being when it cannot be fulfilled.

This last point is important. If it could be shown that to bring into existence a human embryo was, in the sense just defined, to bring into existence a potential person, then it would, in these terms, make good sense to regard the deliberate creation of human embryos for the purposes of research as being ethically more problematic than the use of 'spare' embryos that were a by-product of *in vitro* fertilization that was aimed at treating infertility. (The recommendation, by two members of the Warnock Committee not opposed to human-embryo research as such, that the former practice should be banned thus has a certain logic to it.[13]) By the same token, of course, it would then be rational to prefer techniques that did not generate such spare embryos in the first place, and to prefer those that produced less to those that produced more.

Everything here hinges, however, on the later person actually having existed at the earlier time, albeit bereft of self-awareness and the capacity for reasoned thought and action. That is why the question of when human life begins is crucial and inescapable here. It seems to me that the popular conception, according to which this is the central issue, is correct; and the Warnock Report, and Mary Warnock herself, are quite wrong to reject it. So also, I believe, are they wrong to assume that the question when human life begins has to embody a moral decision. Ultimately, the question of when human life begins must hinge on what constitutes the identity of the kind of beings that we essentially are—which is what I take 'human being' to signify, in common parlance. How far back does my identity extend? What is the earliest point at which there existed something identical with me now? (Not qualitatively, of course, but identical in the sense of the very same individual.) This problem of the identity of human beings is notoriously difficult, philosophically; but it has not generally been thought to turn on any matter of moral decision (which is not to say that no matter of moral decision, given suitable moral premises, can turn on it).

What our identity actually does consist in, as I argued in Chapter 1, partly on philosophical and partly on scientific grounds, is a structural continuity within the brain, specifically within the midbrain and cerebral hemispheres, of those neural structures that underlie continuities of memory, personality, and disposition to thought, feeling, and action. I shall not, however, repeat here the arguments for this conclusion. Suffice it to say that, if I am right, then one is not, in the human embryo of two weeks, confronted with a human being, or even a potential human being, much less a potential person—if by that one means something that has the potential actually itself to be a human being or person. (For the two-week-old embryo does not even have a brain.) So if it is that thought that gives rise to moral qualms in relation to embryo research then such qualms may be dismissed as groundless.

There is, to be sure, another sense in which the embryo clearly is a potential person: it has the potential to give rise to a person. Some people might imagine that this should count for something. But I can see no reason why it should. I strongly suspect, moreover, that it is only their failure to distinguish clearly this weaker sort of potentiality from the stronger kind just discussed that has led people to think that way. Indeed, if it did count for something, then human sperm and ova ought also to have some moral claim on us. It seems to me that those who argue on the basis of this latter, weak sense of potentiality, where to be a potential X is not potentially to be an X, are insufficiently embarrassed by this apparent consequence of their views. It is true, of course, that sperm has to fertilize ovum before development can begin; but why should the separateness of the components be thought to make any difference? (I am reminded of what is popularly supposed to be the case in regard to the atom bomb that the Israelis steadfastly deny that they possess; it has been suggested that they have built and tested the components, but have deliberately refrained from making the final assembly, thus rendering their claim not to have built a nuclear weapon strictly true. But of course if what concerns us is the potentiality for an atomic explosion, that is neither here nor there: the components have that potentiality even in their unassembled state, given that they can readily be assembled.)

What is the practical upshot of all this? I understand that there is not the remotest possibility of the brain structures that (according to the view I favour) are a *sine qua non* of human existence having developed even at six weeks, which is when the embryonic stage of development technically gives way to the foetal stage. Contrast the fact that it is not, at present, possible to keep human embryos alive in the laboratory for more than about ten days. So huge, at present, is the gap between what current technology can accomplish in the way of keeping human embryos alive in the laboratory and the earliest point (perhaps eight to ten weeks) at which the brain might have developed to the extent of being able to support some minimal degree of genuinely mental function—the earliest point, for example, at which it might conceivably be able to suffer—that one might think there was no immediate practical need to legislate a cut-off point on embryo research at all. This is probably true, if one is thinking merely of embryos reared *in vitro*. But of course there is also the problem of regulating research on live *aborted* embryos and foetuses. Although this, strictly speaking, lay outside the Warnock Committee's terms of reference, it is clearly a matter on which legislation is called for; and it would (as the Warnock Report points out[14]) create a curious legal anomaly if the law relating to research on live human embryos and foetuses were to discriminate on the basis of their origin. In any case, the Warnock Committee was clearly expected to set a time limit on human-embryo research, and would doubtless have been considered to be shirking its responsibilities had it failed to do so.

The Report does, in fact, consider the possibility of taking as the cut-off point the onset of 'functional activity' in the central nervous system, remarking, however, that 'in the present state of knowledge the onset of central nervous system functional activity could not be used to define accurately the limit to research, because the timing is not known'.[15] True; but that is no reason for dismissing this as a criterion, if such functional activity is what really counts here. The thing to do, in that case, would be to choose the latest point at which the experts are agreed that such functional activity must be absent.

A working party of the Council for Science and Society, commissioned to deliberate the same range of issues as the Warnock Committee, adopted essentially this approach in their own report—and suggested that six weeks might, from this point of view, be an appropriate limit.[16] I suspect that this may be unduly cautious—and, in any case, functional activity *per se* is not what is crucial, from the point of view I advocate, so much as mental activity. (There is much that goes on in the central nervous system, or even the brain—the mediation of reflexes, for example, and temperature regulation—that has nothing to do with mind.) Nevertheless, six weeks has something to be said for it; setting that as a limit would, as we have seen, be tantamount to saying that research on human embryos was permissible, but research on human foetuses was not. It is sufficiently early, I would have thought, to allay public concern significantly (not, of course, that of supporters of LIFE or the Society for the Protection of the Unborn Child—but then nothing short of a total ban on such research would satisfy them);[17] but sufficiently late not to constrain any research project that would, for the foreseeable future, be technically feasible anyway.

Some might object that, even if there is nothing intrinsically wrong with experimenting on human embryos up to six weeks, to allow experiments that late would be to take a substantial step along what is potentially a very dangerous path. In short, switching to the more familiar metaphor, the proposal is vulnerable to a 'slippery-slope' argument. I believe such an objection to be unfounded in this case (though it isn't exactly a philosophical issue whether it is or not). About the best protection one can have against a slippery slope is to have an enforced limit with a clear point that almost everyone is capable of appreciating. I suggest that a limit, of six weeks say, explained in terms of a 'brain life' criterion, fulfils those conditions. Of course, if that were seen to be the point of the limit, and scientific research subsequently demonstrated that (given the underlying rationale) it was far too early, there might well be pressure from the scientific community to extend it a bit. But that would hardly matter. Anyone could see that the rationale behind the limit would not sanction experimenting on a foetus at a later stage, when it was, say, capable of experiencing pain. Any pressure in that direction, therefore, would have to have quite a different source.

From a purely practical standpoint, fourteen days may well turn out to have been a particularly unfortunate choice of cut-off point, since it is just before the process of differentiation gets under way—the process whereby the cells begin to assume the distinct characters appropriate to skin cells, liver cells, nerve cells and so forth. So far, we have been talking merely of the use of live human embryos for the purposes of scientific research. But they may also turn out to have considerable therapeutic potential. Scandinavian scientists have been experimenting with the use of foetal dopamine-producing cells to treat artificially induced Parkinson's disease in rats. The results have been very promising. Mature dopamine cells, though not rejected, simply do not function in their new setting; but cells taken from live foetuses do. Once the process of differentiation has begun, it may well prove possible to produce from the so-called stem cells that are the ancestors of the cell lines characteristic of various kinds of tissue, all kinds of cell cultures for therapeutic purposes, of which dopamine-producing cells (for those suffering from Parkinson's disease) would be merely one example. It has also been suggested, for instance, that diabetes might be cured by the injection into the pancreas of embryo-derived insulin-producing cells. (Problems of rejection are far less in the case of cells taken from embryos or foetuses.)[18] This is all somewhat speculative; but it would seem to me a tragedy if, as a society, we were to deny people suffering from crippling diseases the possibility of a cure, because we had set the limit on keeping embryos alive in the laboratory at fourteen days, rather than, say, twenty. Admittedly, however, this is said from a philosophical standpoint according to which qualms about the moral status of such embryos are, in any case, totally baseless. It is not intended to sway those who, believing (as I do not) that twenty-day-old human embryos are human beings (or at any rate quasi-human beings), not unreasonably feel that whatever advantages might come from experimenting on or otherwise manipulating them in the laboratory would be purchased at too high a moral price.

There is one other observation in the Report regarding embryo research which seems to me deserving of remark: 'We were agreed' it says 'that the embryo of the human species ought to have a special status and no one should undertake research on human embryos the purposes of which could be achieved by the use of animals or in some other way.'[19] From my point of view there is nothing intrinsically wrong with experimenting on human embryos, given that there is no intention of reimplanting them, and therefore no particular point, ethically speaking, in looking for alternatives. But what I find disturbing here is the suggestion that it would be morally preferable to use live animals. Perhaps all that is meant is that it would be preferable to use animal embryos. If, however, what is meant is that it would be preferable to use mature animals, animals that are aware and capable of suffering, then I recoil at the suggestion. I should have thought that, from any sane point of view, it was far preferable to experiment on a near-microscopic blob of unfeeling protoplasm than a feeling, caring being, albeit of a different species. Indeed, where pain and suffering are concerned, I fail to see what species has to do with it. Suffering of a given intensity is, as far as I can see, no less to be regretted or avoided if it happens to a dog than if it happens to a don. Mary Warnock herself has responded, in a reply to an article by John Harris,[20] to possible charges, in this connection, of 'speciesism' (to use Richard Ryder's infelicitous but convenient term):

It is part of our humanity that we should regard fellow members of the species as in a special relation to ourselves . . . I do not . . . regard a preference for humanity as 'arbitrary', nor do I see it as standing in need of any other justification than that we ourselves are human.[21]

But why could not the white racist argue, in parallel fashion, that he did not see his preference for whites as standing in need of any other justification than that he himself is white? Perhaps Mary Warnock means that morally we ought to feel a special loyalty to members of our own species, just as we would to members of our own family. But this is scarcely a very promising analogy. Family loyalty is based on social ties, not (or at any rate not merely) biological ones. If, on the other hand, it is a question of identification, then I am bound to say that I identify far more strongly with a laboratory rabbit that, like me, sees, feels, and suffers and has a brain, than with a primitive, insensate, and indeed literally brainless clump of cells.

In a sense, of course, all this has been said from a rather narrowly rationalistic standpoint. This is, however, an area where people have strong sentiments and anxieties. The Report declares, in no uncertain terms, that it felt 'bound to take very seriously the feelings expressed in the evidence'.[22] The question thus arises of just how much weight one should give, in this sort of matter, to public sentiment, even if one considers it to be irrational. It is to this question, which has particular application to the second great area of controversy—that of surrogate motherhood —that I now turn.

Morality, freedom, public sentiment, and the law

Mary Warnock was evidently much exercised by the question of what approach, philosophically speaking, the Inquiry should adopt towards the whole enterprise of appraising evidence and deciding on recommendations; of what principles should guide their deliberations. One could, in these matters, adopt what she refers to, both in the Report and elsewhere, as a strict utilitarian approach. A utilitarian, for our purposes, may be thought of as a person who believes that one should strive, in one's actions, to maximize overall benefit and minimize overall harm (however conceived: it is not necessary to assume, as did the classical utilitarians, that happiness, pleasure, or enjoyment are the only things that are of ultimate benefit or that unhappiness, pain, or suffering are the only harms). A strict utilitarian, as Mary Warnock uses the term, is a utilitarian who takes no account, in his moral reckoning, of what Honderich calls morality-dependent harms (or, presumably, though Mary Warnock doesn't say this, of morality-dependent benefits).[23] These are harms that an action causes, not in virtue of its being intrinsically harmful, but because of people's moral attitudes towards it. If, for example, the mere knowledge that a certain activity is taking place causes someone who disapproves of it to be shocked, outraged, disgusted, or saddened, then that would be a morality-dependent harm, in Honderich's sense. Also, if Lord Justice Devlin is right in supposing that some actions, just by virtue of offending against the prevailing moral standards within society, may contribute towards social disintegration,[24] then that too would be a morality-dependent harm, since, if the prevailing standards were other than they are, no such consequence would threaten.

Strict utilitarianism is not very plausible as a theory of morality. Morality-dependent harms are, after all, still harms; why, then, should it be thought appropriate, in one's moral deliberations, to exclude them from consideration? (A girl considering whether to live with her boyfriend ought, one might think, to give some thought to what it would do to Great-Aunt Agatha, with her Victorian upbringing.) The view—at least in its negative aspects—has, however, recommended itself to a number of people as a secondary principle (in Mill's sense[25]), intended only to apply to decisions about legislation (or state interventions generally). Thus understood, it is exemplified by the approach of the Wolfenden Committee on Homosexual Offences and Prostitution,[26] an approach which led them to recommend the legalizing of homosexual acts between consenting adults. The more recent Williams Committee on Obscenity and Film Censorship,[27] adopted a very similar approach in regard to pornography. These committees, both incidentally chaired by philosophers, took the view that the only legitimate basis for using the law to restrict or suppress a given activity was that the activity in question was harmful, in a sense of 'harmful' that would exclude morality-dependent harms. This harm condition, with 'harm' glossed so as to exclude morality-dependent harms, is very explicitly advocated in the Williams Report.[28] (Equally explicit, significantly, is the Report's repudiation of any attempt to use the harm condition to constrain the moral appraisal of actions generally. Bernard Williams is not, in other respects, any particular friend of utilitarianism, strict or otherwise. Nor is the argument he offers, in the Report, for the harm condition ostensibly, at least, a utilitarian one, being based rather on an appeal to the value of individual freedom.[29]) The classic contemporary statement of the opposing viewpoint is that of Lord Justice Devlin, alluded to above, who argued that society has the right to prohibit by law any form of behaviour that the bulk of the populace regards as morally intolerable.[30] This was in a British Academy Address directed specifically at the Wolfenden Report.

Mary Warnock, whose views (as she herself has pointed out in Chapter 7) have much in common with Devlin's, rejects strict utilitarianism as inadequate by itself to guide either our moral thinking in general or the choice of legislation in particular; so also does the Warnock Report.[31] *Pace* Wolfenden and Williams, it is, according to her, not only legitimate but positively obligatory to give weight to people's moral beliefs, to their deeply held moral feelings: morality-dependent harms, she thinks, should figure in the kind of deliberations in which her committee was engaged. That does not mean that the principle of utility, understood as bidding us to maximize morality-independent benefits and minimize morality-independent harms, ought to play no role at all in one's deliberations. On the contrary, it should play a role, according to her. But not in an unconstrained fashion; it is not, as the strict utilitarian would maintain, the only principle to which one should pay heed. A principle of respect for people's moral convictions is needed also to act as 'a counter-argument to the principle of Utility': moral beliefs are to be 'weigh[ed] . . . in the balance against future good'.[32]

This second principle is nowhere very precisely stated. From the examples Mary Warnock uses to illustrate it, however, I take it that she would accept the following gloss. A person's moral beliefs, on a given matter, should be given a weight that is a function of a number of things: their intensity, for example, and their depth (the degree to which the beliefs reflect long-standing, well-entrenched, and relatively fundamental values, ideals, and attitudes) and also the degree to which he or she has a legitimate stake in the matter in question. Mary Warnock thinks, for example, that it would be quite wrong to override the moral feelings of the (biological) mother with regard to the use of a spare embryo or aborted foetus for research purposes.[33] A recommendation to that effect appears in the Report.[34] The point, I take it, is that being the mother (or father—the Report says consent must, wherever possible, be obtained from the couple) gives her a legitimate stake in the matter of the use to which the embryo or foetus is put, adequate respect for which entails giving her a power of veto over any proposal to experiment on it. In a wider context, however, Mary Warnock clearly thinks that we all have a legitimate interest in the kind of society in which we live. Thus any form of behaviour which may affect the character of the society and, in particular, which bears on the future of social institutions such as the family, is something in which any citizen may be said to have a legitimate stake. No doubt the stake that any arbitrary citizen may be said to have in the—not palpably harmful—behaviour of an arbitrary fellow member of the society, of which he happens nevertheless strongly to disapprove, will, taken in isolation, be relatively small. But when the bulk of people in a society feel the same way, and the proliferation of such behaviour could make for a qualitative and non-trivial change in the society's moral aspect, this sort of legitimate concern can, in aggregate, create a moral pressure which demands to be taken seriously. So it is, Mary Warnock believes, with the widespread concern currently felt about the growing practice of surrogate motherhood, and in particular the setting up of commercial surrogacy agencies.

Bernard Williams and, of course, John Stuart Mill[35] would see in this line of thought the spectre of a 'tyranny of the majority' (in de Tocqueville's phrase)—the possibility of individual freedom being sacrificed on the altar of majority prejudice. The desirability of avoiding that is, in essence, the Williams Report's main argument for the harm condition, with its associated exclusion of morality-dependent harms. If the argument were sound, it would constitute a decisive objection to the view just outlined— the view that underlies the Warnock Report. But it is not sound, in my opinion. I think the argument underestimates the philosophical resources of a pluralistic scheme of values such as Mary Warnock is, in effect, advocating. To be sure, allowing a principle of respect for people's moral beliefs to operate in an unconstrained fashion could in principle have the most illiberal or otherwise repugnant consequences. (Hideous things have been done, over the years, to racial, religious, and political minorities in deference to the moral opinions of a bigoted majority.) But Mary Warnock herself explicitly says that a principle of respect for people's moral beliefs is to be constrained both by considerations of utility— benefit and harm—on the one hand, and by a respect for individual liberty on the other: 'where the question is whether, or to what extent, the law should be interventionist, in order to protect people's moral scruples' she says '[l]aws have to balance liberty against offence'.[36] No one is suggesting that a principle of respect for the prevailing morality be allowed to ride roughshod over all other considerations.

It is arguable, indeed, that there is no need to appeal to a separate principle of individual liberty to block what would other- wise be unacceptably illiberal consequences of Mary Warnock's principle of respect for moral beliefs. For it could plausibly be argued that a principle of respect for individual liberty is effectively already contained within her principle. What we would have, on the view I have in mind, is a single unitary principle according to which people have a right to order things, to shape the world and what happens within it, to the extent that it is theirs to shape, in accordance with their conception of the good.[37] When we think of this principle in relation to people's ordering of their own lives, we speak of individual liberty or personal autonomy; when we think of it at a collective level, at the level of an entire community, then we speak of democracy and so forth. It is perhaps no accident, and implies no real ambiguity, that the phrase 'self-determination' is used as a synonym for both. From this point of view, there is a built-in brake on the imposition of majority moral opinion upon the conduct of individuals. If the underlying principle is just that people be allowed to order their affairs, or have them ordered, in accordance with their moral convictions, then beyond a certain point it can make no sense to claim that individual freedom may legitimately be constrained in the name of the prevailing morality. For any gain to the principle at the collective level will be cancelled by a corresponding loss, of greater magnitude, at the individual level. Self-determination will effectively be at war with itself.

Surrogacy

There is more that needs to be said on the proper role of public sentiment in helping to determine social policy and legislation. It is perhaps better said, however, not in the abstract, but in relation to the particular issue, out of those dealt with in the Report, on which it appears to have most bearing: surrogate motherhood.

The terms 'surrogate motherhood' or 'surrogacy' are used to cover two importantly distinct practices. In one, the male partner of a couple provides sperm, which is then used to inseminate a woman, the surrogate, so that she can conceive a child, carry it to term, and then hand it over to the couple. Here the surrogate mother is also the genetic mother of the resulting child. In the second sort of case, a woman has one or more eggs removed from her ovaries, one of which is then fertilized *in vitro*, usually with sperm from her husband. The resulting embryo is then transferred to the womb of the surrogate mother, again with the hope that she will bear a child which she will later hand over. Here the surrogate mother is not the genetic mother. As far as I am aware, no actual child has yet been born by the latter method; but there are no technical obstacles to it. The normal assumption is that couples or single women would resort to these methods only if they believed themselves to be unable (or unable safely) to have children by normal means. But that is not necessarily the case. A woman might resort to surrogacy in order to avoid the disruption to her career that pregnancy might involve, or even (especially if she was a model, say, or a film star) to avoid the risk of harming her figure. The Warnock Committee was unanimous in finding surrogacy for convenience morally unacceptable.[38] So do I, and though it may be an interesting philosophical exercise to try to work out just why this seems so obviously objectionable, it is one I leave to others.

As the law stands at present, there is nothing to prevent people entering into a private surrogacy arrangement of the first kind, with the couple adopting the resulting child. But it seems improbable that any court of law would regard a surrogacy contract as having any legal force.[39] The Warnock Report recommends that such private arrangements continue to be legal, but that surrogacy contracts be made legally unenforceable as a matter of statute.[40] This would mean that no surrogate mother could be forced to give up the child; though it might still be possible for the commissioning couple to retrieve any money that had changed hands by going through the civil courts.

What has given rise to most public concern are the activities in this country of (American-run) commercial surrogacy agencies. The Warnock Committee was unanimous that commercial agencies should be banned completely—that operating such an agency should be made a criminal offence. The Committee was, however, divided on the question whether non-profit-making agencies should, subject to careful regulation, be permitted to offer a surrogacy service. A minority thought they should.[41] In the end, however, a majority of the Committee favoured making it a criminal offence for anyone other than the commissioning couple and the surrogate mother herself (even, say, the family doctor) knowingly to assist in establishing a surrogate pregnancy.[42]

Were these recommendations to be passed into law, the legal status of surrogacy, in this country, would be closely analogous to that of prostitution. How, then, was the Warnock Committee led to recommend such sweeping legislation? Were their reasons sound?

It would be difficult, I think, to make out a convincing case even against commercial surrogacy agencies, simply on the basis of their doing palpable, morality-independent harm. Who, after all, is harmed? If all goes to plan, the agency and the surrogate mother end up richer, with the added satisfaction of having brought happiness to others, a couple end up poorer but with a much longed-for child, and a child gains a life, presumably with adoring parents. It appears that statistically that is actually the way it turns out, more often than not. (A surrogacy agency in Los Angeles, by dint of careful screening of would-be surrogates, claims to have arranged twenty-six such transactions without a single hitch.[43]) Sometimes, to be sure, things go badly wrong. The surrogate mother changes her mind, wants to keep the baby, and there are recriminations and anguish all round. There may also, of course, be emotional hazards, both for the surrogate mother herself, who may feel guilt in consequence of giving up the child (though it would seem that she had a lot less reason to feel that than a woman who had, say, had a late abortion), or to the child, who might well, on learning the truth, suffer problems of identity. My colleague, Robert Elmore, has raised also the possible problem of what he calls 'the precious child syndrome'; it may not always be good for a child to have parents that wanted parenthood so much and achieved it with such difficulty. But that, of course, is just as likely to apply in the case of the IVF child, or, indeed, in other perfectly 'normal' cases.

Mary Warnock has stated publicly that possible hazards to the child were a major influence on her Committee's recommendations (though this is not made clear in the Report itself).[44] But even if there were solid reasons for fearing for the child's welfare here— and at the moment this is sheer speculation—there is something illogical, on the face of it, in using this as an argument against surrogacy. For a child born as the result of a surrogacy arrange- ment would not otherwise have existed at all; it is difficult to believe that the problems it faces are likely to be so severe that it would rather not have been born at all, or even so severe that others are likely to end up wishing that. (This sort of point is one that Derek Parfit has been urging for years and one which is made, in relation to embryo donation, by Peter Singer and Deane Wells.[45]) In any case, life is beset by pitfalls, and beyond a certain point it is no purpose of government to cushion people against these—only, perhaps, to try to ensure that people are made adequately aware of the risks they may be running. For all its risks, surrogacy is, judging by what one reads, no worse a bet than love or marriage; and we do not ban commercial dating agencies and marriage bureaux.

Surrogacy is sometimes seen as representing a threat to the marriage relationship or to the institution of the family. Mary Warnock, in her contribution to this volume, cites the argument that it may involve a 'damaging' 'intrusion of a third person into the marriage-relation', a point that is made also in the Report.[46] Precisely what sort of damage is being envisaged is unclear, or even whether this is supposed to be a utilitarian argument at all: perhaps it is thought intrinsically damaging that a third party become involved, in the way that the surrogate mother does (or might), in the lives of the commissioning couple. But this hypothetical, if not wholly notional, harm counts for little, I should have thought, beside the known fact that infertility itself can place a very heavy, sometimes intolerable, strain upon a marriage.

That surrogacy somehow threatens to change or undermine the family is an objection that has been urged by a number of people, for example by Keith Ward, Professor of Moral and Social Theology at King's College, London.[47] But, on reflection, this hardly seems plausible. In the first place, all the evidence goes to suggest that the family is one of the most robust and resilient things going, sociologically speaking; even deliberate attempts to move away from the traditional family, as in some of the early Israeli kibbutzim, or the communes of the sixties and early seventies, have met with negligible success. Secondly, a normal family is precisely what those who resort to surrogacy are, after all, trying to achieve—a normal family being one in which there are children. And finally, it will only ever be a very small proportion of couples that would have any reason to seek surrogate mothers: namely, those couples in which the woman is (a) unable to have babies by normal means, and (b) cannot be helped by other treatments for infertility. As new techniques such as IVF and egg donation become more widely available, the number, already very small, is likely to fall still further. The scale on which surrogacy is likely to be practised is never going to be sufficient to have any impact on the institution of the family or marriage in general.

But, as we have seen, it is, in any case, Mary Warnock's firm conviction that an issue such as this cannot be settled merely by reference to utilitarian considerations of this sort. This is made clear in the Foreword to the Report:

A strict utilitarian would suppose that, given certain procedures, it would be possible to calculate their benefits and their costs. Future advantages, therapeutic and scientific, should be weighed against present and future harm. However, even if such a calculation were possible, it could not provide a final or verifiable answer whether it is right that such procedures should be carried out. There would still remain the possibility that they were unacceptable, whatever their long-term benefits were supposed to be. Moral questions, such as those with which we have been concerned are, by definition, questions that involve not only a calculation of consequences, but also strong sentiments with regard to the nature of the proposed activities themselves.

We were therefore bound to take very seriously the feelings expressed in the evidence.[48]

What is being urged, here, is a conception of morality which will allow us, indeed oblige us, as the strict utilitarian conception does not, to take seriously the kind of intuitive or emotive moral responses that the ordinary person (Devlin's 'man on the Clapham omnibus') actually expresses. Mary Warnock has, by her own account, been much influenced here by the views of Stuart Hampshire, particularly as expressed in his Leslie Green Lecture, 'Morality and Pessimism', which is quoted with approval (though without explicit attribution) in the Foreword to the Warnock Report.[49] It may be instructive, in this context, to consider some observations that have actually been offered, by non-philosophers, in regard to commercially organized surrogacy—all, as it happens, garnered from the tabloid Press, and the first three coming from Members of Parliament. (The occasion for the MPs' remarks was the announcement by Mr Bill Handel, on his arrival in Britain, that he was offering British couples the chance to have surrogate pregnancies arranged at the clinic he runs in California.)

'We don't want baby-farm clinics in Britain where one woman has a baby for another out of money and greed.' (Mrs Anna McCurley, whose Bill to outlaw commercial surrogacy agencies failed for lack of time in the 1983–4 Parliamentary session)

'These are callous and coldblooded transactions which should be stopped.' (Mr Peter Bruinvels)

'immoral, distasteful and bordering on the disgusting . . . reeking of stud farm mentality . . .' (Mr Nicholas Winterton)[50]

'no better than prostitution' (the brother of surrogate mother Mrs Kim Cotton)[51]

Such remarks clearly fail to make the grade, as serious contributions to the discussion, if the only rationally defensible approach to the issue is thought to be a careful weighing of harms and benefits. As Hampshire says,

There is a model of rational reflection which depends upon a contrast between the primitive moral response of an uneducated man, and of an uneducated society, and the comparatively detached arguments of the sophisticated moralist, who discounts his intuitive responses as being prejudices inherited from an uncritical past . . . empirical calculation succeeds a priori prejudice, and the calculation of consequences is reason.[52]

Common-sense moral judgements hardly ever conform to this model of rationality: far from making any explicit appeal to consequences, they usually present actions or practices as worthy of admiration or condemnation because they exemplify or fail to exemplify certain virtues, vices, worthy or unworthy motives, or a style of going about things, a form of life even, which we are expected to think in themselves decent or praiseworthy, base or contemptible. And even these connections are not always ones we are capable of drawing explicitly: in that sense they may well be mere 'intuitive responses'. For Hampshire our judgements are none the worse for being like that. He does not explicitly consider the 'sophisticated moralist's' rejoinder that, where such judgements are defensible, it is only because thinking in these terms happens to be the most effective strategy for promoting overall utility; but doubtless he would consider it inadequate, and perhaps philistine. The proper way to regard moral prohibitions is, he thinks, not merely as being conditional upon their having certain beneficial consequences, but as constituting 'a kind of grammar of conduct, showing the elements out of which any fully respectworthy conduct, as one conceives it, must be built'.[53]

It is this conception, or something very close to it, that informs much of Mary Warnock's own thinking. And to Hampshire she adds a touch of Hume (also quoted in the Foreword to the Report): at some sufficiently basic level of our moral thinking, feelings are all we have to go on anyway. Reason, in the end, is the slave of the passions. Mary Warnock clearly had to struggle to get this across to her Committee:

It is difficult to persuade members of committees that feelings or sentiments can have a central role to play in decision-making. Such people tend to believe that a moral judgement must be rational, or else it must be based on religious dogma. Otherwise it will not count as a properly moral judgement. They find it shocking to accept that, as Hume put it, 'morality is more properly felt than judged of'. Yet I believe that it is to offend against the concept of morality itself to refuse to take moral feelings or sentiments into account in decision-making.[54]

Whether this conception of morality is indeed the correct one is something that I shall not here attempt to adjudicate. Suffice it to say that it seems to me at least an open question whether the intuitive thinking of common-sense morality might not ultimately be given a rational justification in consequentialist terms. This is certainly what Hare believes;[55] and nothing that Hampshire or Warnock says seems to constitute a refutation of this claim. Utilitarianism is, at base, a theory about aims, not about strategy. For all kinds of reasons, the overall goal of maximizing benefits and minimizing harm may often be more effectively furthered by adopting a rule or prohibition on the strength of the judged usual consequences of observing it (or developing, in oneself or others, some trait of character or disposition towards immediate judgement or action, on the strength of the judged consequences of possessing it) and then obeying the rule unquestioningly in most contexts (or simply acting as one's character or 'intuition' prompts), rather than by thinking out anew how to act on every occasion.

The power of this distinction between aims and strategy is not always adequately appreciated by critics of utilitarianism. Mary Warnock cites with approval Stuart Hampshire's observation that the acceptance of utilitarianism 'may well lead to a brutal counting of heads, and an insensitivity to the kinds of inhibitions and scruples which are at the centre of morality' (Warnock's words, not Hampshire's).[56] So it may. But there is no particular reason for the utilitarian to be discomfited by that. For either these inhibitions and scruples are themselves helping to further the good, as the utilitarian conceives it, or they are not. If they are not, then a loosening of their grip is, from his point of view, to be welcomed as a liberation. But if they are, and it is really true that thinking, constantly, in explicitly utilitarian terms would have the effect of undermining them, then all that follows is that this is not what a utilitarian appraisal, at the level of policy, would recommend: it is not, after all, the optimum strategy for maximizing benefit and minimizing harm.

Be that as it may, one thing that must be stressed is that even intuitive morality is constrained by canons of rationality. To quote Hampshire again,

A reflective, critical scrutiny of moral claims is compatible . . . with an overriding concern for a record of un-monstrous and respectworthy conduct, and of action that has never been mean or inhuman; and it may follow an assessment of the worth of persons which is not to be identified only with a computation of consequences and effects.[57]

Mary Warnock says that 'moral feelings should be respected even if they seem 'unreasonable' or 'silly'.[58] Perhaps they should— sometimes, and to some degree. But this does not follow from the conception of morality that she favours; nor does it obviously follow from the principle of collective self-determination that was defended above. It is perfectly possible to think that people's moral views should count for something and yet also think that, if it is to deserve to be taken seriously, a moral view, however widely shared, must meet certain minimal standards of rationality. This was the line taken by Dworkin in response to Devlin's attack, referred to earlier, on the Wolfenden Committee's recommendation that homosexual acts between consenting adults be legalized. Devlin's own stress on the importance of moral feelings, especially feelings of 'reprobation', 'indignation', 'intolerance', and 'disgust', parodied by Hart as the view that something is immoral, by society's lights, 'if the thought of it makes the man on the Clapham omnibus sick',[59] prompted Dworkin to write: 'What is shocking and wrong is not his idea that the community's morality counts, but his idea of what counts as the community's morality.'[60] Right or wrong, it is an idea that Mary Warnock would appear to share. But is it wrong?

This is not, perhaps, the kind of question that admits of an unqualified 'Yes' or 'No'. On the one hand there is obviously something right about Dworkin's insistence that we are entitled to 'test the credentials' of an apparent moral consensus—to ask whether it may simply be an expression of 'prejudice, rationalization, or personal aversion' or, as Hart says, 'ignorance, superstition or misunderstanding'.[61] But on the other hand it is not clear that we are entitled to discount entirely views that are found wanting in this regard: there is something right, also, in Devlin's dictum that society's morality should be gauged by the standards of 'the reasonable . . . not . . . the rational man'.[62] We do not let lunatics vote, but for the rest we do not feel it necessary or desirable to 'test the credentials' of the political preferences expressed at the polls. Why should society's moral preferences be regarded differently? (Also, I sense a certain special pleading, especially in Dworkin. Dworkin, I think, has the problem that anyone has, if he wishes simultaneously to be a populist and a liberal, when he finds that the public have illiberal views. The standards of rationality which he insists that a supposed moral opinion must meet in order to be regarded genuinely as such are perhaps just a little too conveniently tailored to filter out views that would offend the liberal conscience.)

There are two key points to be made here. First, we believe in political leadership; most of us believe that those we elect to positions of power and influence should behave as representatives, in Burke's sense,[63] not just as delegates. They are, after all, elected for their supposed judgement and we should expect them to exercise it. And what goes for elected representatives presumably ought, logically, to apply *a fortiori* to their appointed advisors. Respect for people's moral views ought to be one of the values to which they pay heed, in making their decisions; but it is one consideration among others. We would surely expect them —and this is the second point—to ask, when faced with evidence of public opinion, whether the expressed view really followed, given the facts, from people's underlying ideals. For people's basic values are deserving of respect quite as much as are their specific opinions on specific topics. And, what is more, to the extent that their specific opinions are grounded in factual mis-apprehension or muddled thinking, they are less likely to survive the test of time. It would be irresponsible for any legislator to legislate today on the basis of opinions which he had good reason to suppose would be different tomorrow. Opinions do shift, and sometimes do so in response to considerations of reason and sometimes, indeed, in response to enlightened legislation. (It is worth noting, in this connection, that the public abhorrence towards homosexual acts to which Devlin was responding, is, according to the latest opinion polls, no longer felt by a majority in this country.[64])

In this spirit, then, let us subject to 'reflective, critical scrutiny' the sorts of (not ostensibly utilitarian) considerations that seem actually to move most critics of surrogate motherhood.

Since a majority of the Warnock Committee apparently wanted to place surrogacy in a similar position to that of prostitution, it is perhaps worth asking, to begin with, whether it has anything im-portantly in common with prostitution. Prostitution is generally regarded as essentially degrading to the prostitute herself, and frequently to her clients also. And it is commonly thought to involve exploitation, again not necessarily just of the prostitute herself, but quite possibly of her clients. Something is degrading, I take it, if it is inconsistent with human dignity; though quite what that means is not easy to explain. To exploit someone, on the other hand, is to use them in a way that is unjust or unfair. These concepts are clearly connected, in the present context. What makes one person's use of another a case of exploitation may, in part at least, be the fact that what one is getting the other to do is something that degrades that person.

Prostitution, I suggested, is essentially degrading. It is impos-sible to imagine a genuine case of prostitution which is not degrading to some extent, even though it may, all things considered, be morally admirable (as with the resistance worker who sets up as a prostitute in order to gain valuable information from soldiers and officials of the occupying power). Surrogacy, I submit, is not essentially degrading. There is nothing in the least degrading in the actions of a woman who, through love for her childless sister, agrees to be inseminated with her sister's husband's sperm, so that she can give her and her husband the baby they long for. Here it is not, as with the resistance worker, a case of the intrinsically degrading character of the act somehow being outweighed by other ennobling features; there is simply nothing degrading about it. Nor, if the woman freely offers her services to her sister, and is in no way pressured into it, need there be any exploitation here. (I have little doubt, from what I have heard her say, that Mary Warnock would agree with that.) So we have established something important; if surrogacy is degrading, if it involves exploitation, this will be a consequence of contingent, in principle avoidable, features of the practice.

Motive (or presumed motive) is obviously a crucial factor here. The fact that it is done for gain, usually monetary gain, is what makes prostitution what it is and what makes it degrading: it serves to turn the sexual act into something squalid. (For that reason, the resistance worker would, in a moral sense, be prostituting herself even if she was just sleeping with enemy soldiers, solely for the purpose of gaining information, without actually being paid by them.) One may be tempted to think that pregnancy must likewise be made squalid by the introduction of a financial motive. But that does not necessarily follow. Sex for money or gain is degrading mainly because the motive serves to cheapen and distort the character of the relationship between the people involved in the sexual act. (Typically, indeed, there is no relationship beyond that of customer and purveyor.) Pregnancy, however, does not involve a relationship in anything like the same sense. It is thus far from obvious that it is in danger of being cheapened or rendered squalid by the introduction of a financial motive, in the same way or to the same extent that the sexual act is. Doubtless many mothers-to-be think of themselves as having a relationship with their babies; but it is a very one-sided and opaque relationship, and the baby's side of it, until it is born, is likely to be sublimely unaffected by its mother's motives.

A rather different reason why surrogacy may be thought to be degrading is that it is somehow thought of as dehumanizing. People sometimes express their moral distaste for surrogacy by drawing an analogy, not so much with the prostitute as with the brood mare, as witness Nicholas Winterton's 'stud farm' analogy. But the main point about the brood mare is that she is simply a cog in a commercial machine and that what she is made to do, while it may exploit her own instincts, is not something she chooses but a form of life that is imposed from without. To treat a woman like that would indeed be dehumanizing. The surrogate mother, however, does after all choose to be that. Mary Warnock suggests in Chapter 7 that, notwithstanding that it is a matter (presumably) of free choice, the surrogate mother is, all the same, being 'used for an end that is not her own' and that this may be morally objectionable. The Warnock Report makes the same point.[65] There is a sense, of course, in which many, perhaps most, forms of employment involve using the employee for an end which is not his own. But we do not, as a rule, think that that automatically makes such forms of employment degrading or dehumanizing; it is simply an inevitable concomitant of working for others. It might, however, be thought to become degrading when it touches a person as intimately as pregnancy does. The kind of 'distancing' that we can all engage in in relation to many of our activities is not something that a woman can readily accomplish in relation to her own reproductive functions; and it is not something we would wish her to do, or morally approve of her doing, even if she could accomplish it. With surrogacy, one might say, the Marxist concept of 'alienated labour' takes on a whole new significance!

If that is the key point, however, there is no reason for a woman who volunteers to be a surrogate to feel degraded or dehumanized, where she actually identifies with the end, and derives satisfaction from the thought that she is bringing happiness to another couple. In this sense, surrogacy can be wholly redeemed, it seems to me, by the spirit in which it is carried out, if the spirit is one of generosity. And I don't see that that is incompatible with the surrogate mother's being paid reasonable compensation for the risks she undertakes and the sacrifices she has to make.

The practice of surrogacy as such has, it seems to me, suffered a kind of guilt by association with the rather crass cashing-in by commercial agencies that has recently been attracting such widespread publicity. People feel, very naturally, that the miracle of birth somehow becomes tainted by being made the subject of a commercial transaction. They don't wish to see the child being reduced to the level of a commodity. This sort of feeling, which bears on the very character of the society in which we live, is precisely of the kind that ought to be respected, in the name of collective self-determination, even by those who happen not to share it, or who judge it to be irrational. But it is far from clear that the practice of surrogacy in general should be allowed to be tarred with the same brush. One consideration which has evidently influenced the Warnock Committee is the thought that, even with a non-profit agency, one would almost certainly have to pay a fee to the surrogate mother. While there may be some women who would be willing to have babies for total strangers as an act of pure altruism, it seems likely that they would be very few and far between. In general one would have reason to be suspicious of the motives (and even mental stability) of a woman who volunteered her services on these terms, without expecting any financial reward. No doubt there are those who will think that the mere fact that money changes hands somehow puts the whole enterprise beyond the pale. But, soberly regarded, that is surely an over-reaction—indicative, perhaps, of a puritanism about money that is peculiarly British, largely absurd, and probably hypocritical. If indeed it is true that the majority of people would be opposed even to properly regulated non-profit agencies offering a surrogacy service (and I doubt whether, in this regard, the evidence submitted to the Inquiry is likely to have been wholly representative, given that the indignant tend to shout loudest), I suspect that this is because they have not really clearly distinguished, in their minds, between this and the activities of commercial agencies.[66] Indeed, the kind of coverage which surrogacy has been receiving in the popular press has hardly been conducive to clear thinking about this issue at all. In short, to echo Dworkin, I would doubt the credentials of any purported consensus on this matter. Good political judgement is frequently a matter of knowing when one should follow and when one should attempt to lead public opinion. To throw out surrogacy agencies altogether with the dirty bathwater of unwanted commercialization might or might not be a victory for public opinion. But it would almost certainly be a defeat for good sense.

There is one final point, which was put to me by Ian Kennedy. Suppose, contrary to what I have been arguing, one were to conclude that surrogacy, even under the auspices of non-profit agencies, was after all morally objectionable and therefore to be firmly discouraged. Even so, why should it be thought to follow that one should make the facilitation of a surrogate pregnancy a crime? The courts and the police, one might think, already have enough on their plates. Might it not be just as effective, and far more appropriate, to try to get the relevant professional bodies to write a ban on knowingly helping to establish surrogate pregnancies into their respective codes of professional conduct? This could include, not only doctors, nurses, and midwives, but also solicitors, who might be called upon to help draft surrogacy agreements. The criminal law is, arguably, a blunt instrument which should be employed only as a last resort.

Since much of what I have been saying has been critical, let me end by saying that there is, in the Report, much that is to be admired. Indeed, it is in many ways a model of what a government report should be: lucid, fair-minded, and, above all, highly readable—with none of the ponderous, indigestible prose that is a feature of so many reports. Moreover, Mary Warnock herself, as Chairman, has done an altogether remarkable job in welding the evidently very disparate views of her Committee into a philosophically coherent whole. The Report deserves to be widely read. That said, I hope that people will regard it as a starting-point for serious discussion of the issues with which it deals, not as bringing the public debate to a close.

9 ON TELLING PATIENTS THE TRUTH

ROGER HIGGS

That honesty should be an important issue for debate in medical circles may seem bizarre. Nurses and doctors are usually thought of as model citizens. Outside the immediate field of health care, when a passport is to be signed, a reference given, or a special allowance made by a government welfare agency, a nurse's or doctor's signature is considered a good warrant, and false certification treated as a serious breach of professional conduct. Yet at the focus of medical activity or skill, at the bedside or in the clinic, when patient meets professional there is often doubt. Is the truth being told?

Many who are unfamiliar with illness and its treatment may well be forgiven for wondering if this doubt has not been exaggerated. It is as if laundry men were to discuss the merits of clean clothes, or fishmongers of refrigeration. But those with experience, either as patients or professionals, will immediately recognize the situation. Although openness is increasingly practised, there is still uncertainty in the minds of many doctors or nurses faced with communicating bad news; as for instance when a test shows up an unexpected and probably incurable cancer, or when meeting the gaze of a severely ill child, or answering the questions of a mother in mid-pregnancy whose unborn child is discovered to be badly handicapped. What should be said? There can be few who have not, on occasions such as these, told less than the truth. Certainly the issue is a regular preoccupation of nurses and doctors in training. Why destroy hope? Why create anxiety, or something worse? Isn't it 'First, do no harm'?[1]

The concerns of the patient are very different. For many, fear of the unknown is the worst disease of all, and yet direct information seems so hard to obtain. The ward round goes past quickly, unintelligible words are muttered—was I supposed to hear and understand? In the surgery the general practitioner signs his prescription pad and clearly it's time to be gone. Everybody is too busy saving lives to give explanations. It may come as a shock to learn that it is policy, not just pressure of work, that prevents a patient learning the truth about himself. If truth is the first casualty, trust must be the second. 'Of course they wouldn't say, especially if things were bad,' said the elderly woman just back from out-patients, 'they've got that Oath, haven't they?' She had learned to expect from doctors, at the best, silence; at the worst, deception. It was part of the system, an essential ingredient, as old as Hippocrates. However honest a citizen, it was somehow part of the doctor's job not to tell the truth to his patient.

These reactions, from both patient and doctor, are most commonly encountered when there is news to communicate of a relatively insidious and life-threatening disease like cancer. Often a collusion seems to be set up, preventing openness on either side. A 45-year-old woman, married with one son of nine, was diagnosed as having acute myeloid leukaemia, and in spite of the treatment was dying in hospital. In response to enquiries, her practitioner was told that she had asked no questions, and didn't want to know anything. The practice nurse, whom she knew, visited the ward. After half an hour the patient burst into tears, desperate to discuss what was going to happen to her son when she died.

However harrowing these occasions, it is easier to decide what to do when the ultimate outcome is clear. It may be much more difficult to know what to say when the future is less certain, such as in the first episode of what is probably multiple sclerosis, or when a patient is about to undergo a mutilating operation. But even in work outside hospital, where such dramatic problems arise less commonly, whether to tell the truth and how much to tell can still be a regular issue. How much should this patient know about the side effects of his drugs? An elderly man sits weeping in an old people's home, and the healthy but exhausted daughter wants the doctor to tell her father that she's medically unfit to have him back. The single mother wants a certificate to say that she is unwell so that she can stay at home to look after her sick child. A colleague is often drunk on duty, and is making mistakes. A husband with venereal disease wants his wife to be treated without her knowledge. An outraged father demands to know if his teenage daughter has been put on the pill. A mother comes in with a child to have a boil lanced. 'Please tell him it won't hurt.' A former student writes from abroad needing to complete his professional experience and asks for a reference for a job he didn't do.[2] Whether the issue is large or small, the truth is at stake. What should the response be?

Discussion of the apparently more dramatic situations may provide a good starting point. Recently a small group of medical students, new to clinical experience, were hotly debating what a patient with cancer should be told. One student maintained strongly that the less said to the patient the better. Others disagreed. When asked whether there was any group of patients they could agree should never be told the truth about a life-threatening illness, the students chose children, and agreed that they would not speak openly to children under six. When asked to try to remember what life was like when they were six, one student replied that he remembered how his mother had died when he was that age. Suddenly the student who had advocated non-disclosure became animated. 'That's extraordinary. My mother died when I was six too. My father said she'd gone away for a time, but would come back soon. One day he said she was coming home again. My younger sister and I were very excited. We waited at the window upstairs until we saw his car drive up. He got out and helped a woman out of the car. Then we saw. It wasn't mum. I suppose I never forgave him—or her, really.'[3]

It is hard to know with whom to sympathize in this sad tale. But its stark simplicity serves to highlight some essential points. First, somehow more clearly than in the examples involving patients, not telling the truth is seen for what it really is. It is, of course, quite possible, and very common in clinical practice, for doctors (or nurses) to engage in deliberate deceit without actually *saying* anything they believe to be false. But, given the special responsibilities of the doctor, and the relationship of trust that exists beween him and his patient, one could hardly argue that this was morally any different from telling outright lies. Surely it is the *intention* that is all important. We may be silent, tactful, or reserved, but if we intend to deceive, what we are doing is tantamount to lying. The debate in ward or surgery is suddenly stood on its head. The question is no longer 'Should we tell the truth?' but 'What justification is there for telling a lie?' This relates to the second important point, that medical ethics are part of general morality, and not a separate field of their own with their own rules. Unless there are special justifications, health-care professionals are working within the same moral constraints as lay people. A lie is a lie wherever told and whoever tells it.

But do doctors have a special dispensation from the usual principles that guide the conduct of our society? It is widely felt that on occasion they do, and such a dispensation is as necessary to all doctors as freedom from the charge of assault is to a surgeon. But if it is impossible to look after ill patients and always be open and truthful, how can we balance this against the clear need for truthfulness on all other occasions? If deception is like a medicine to be given in certain doses in certain cases, what guidance exists about its administration?

My elderly patient reflected the widely held view that truth-telling, or perhaps withholding, was part of the tradition of medicine enshrined in its oaths and codes. Although the writer of the 'Decorum' in the Hippocratic corpus advises physicians of the danger of telling patients about the nature of their illness '. . . for many patients through this cause have taken a turn for the worse',[4] the Oath itself is completely silent on this issue. This extraordinary omission is continued through all the more modern codes and declarations. The first mention of veracity as a principle is to be found in the American Medical Association's 'Principles of Ethics' of 1980, which states that the physician should 'deal honestly with patients and colleagues and strive to expose those physicians deficient in character or competence, or who engage in fraud and deception'.[5] Despite the difficulties of the latter injunction, which seems in some way to divert attention from the basic need for honest communication with the patient, here at last is a clear statement. This declaration signally fails, however, to provide the guidance that we might perhaps have expected for the professional facing his or her individual dilemma.

The reticence of these earlier codes is shared, with some important exceptions, by medical writing elsewhere. Until recently most of what had been usefully said could be summed up by the articles of medical writers such as Thomas Percival, Worthington Hooker, Richard Cabot, and Joseph Collins, which show a wide scatter of viewpoints but do at least confront the problems directly.[6] There is, however, one widely quoted statement by Lawrence Henderson, writing in the *New England Journal of Medicine* in 1955.[7] 'It is meaningless to speak of telling the truth, the whole truth and nothing but the truth to a patient . . . because it is . . . a sheer impossibility . . . Since telling the truth is impossible, there can be no sharp distinction between what is true and what is false.' Unfortunately, Henderson's analysis embodies a major and important error. This feeling of 'unknowableness', the 'soap in the bath' quality of truth as a concept has fascinated many, and has become a central issue of epistemology (the philosophical theory of knowledge), attracting practical, clever, kind, and thoughtful people away by its siren song. 'Truth is a river that is always splitting up into arms that reunite,' said Cyril Connolly. 'Islanded between the arms, the inhabitants argue for a lifetime as to which is the main river.'[8] A superficial understanding of modern physics, with Heisenberg's fascinating uncertainty principle, has helped to confuse medical thinkers further.[9] The more precise our knowledge of the positions of subatomic particles, the less precise, in consequence, must be our knowledge of their velocities and vice versa. If we can never know the whole truth in any situation, what need have we to struggle to think whether to tell or not to tell?

But we must not allow ourselves to be confused, as Henderson was, and as so many others have been, by a failure to distinguish between truth, the abstract concept, of which we shall always have an imperfect grasp, and *telling* the truth, where the intention is all important. Whether or not we can ever fully grasp or express the whole picture, whether we know ultimately what the truth really is, we must speak truthfully, and intend to convey what we understand, or we shall lie. In Sissela Bok's words 'The moral question of whether you are lying or not is not *settled* by establishing the truth or falsity of what you say. In order to settle the question, we must know whether you *intend your statement to mislead*.'[10]

Although epistemology and ethics overlap, the distinction must be made before we can proceed. It is interesting how much primacy has been given to epistemology by modern thinkers, and how often moral issues have taken second place. Perhaps this explains why, until recently, practising health professionals have felt they have had so little help from philosophers. The pendulum may be in danger of swinging too far the other way, and now perhaps too much may be expected from philosophy.[11] However, for medical or nursing practitioners the essentially practical nature of the task has to be kept in mind. Scepticism has its place, but applied morality is the field in which they labour, in which so much is left to be done. For the spade-work we often have to return to classical or medieval thinkers.

Plato was among the first to suggest that falsehood should be available to physicians as 'medicine' for the good of patients (but not to lawyers who should have no part in it!). Sidgwick followed him in arguing that lies to invalids and children could sometimes be justified as being in the best interests of those deceived.[12] But by and large, most early philosophers have looked to truthfulness as fundamental to trust between men. There is a division of opinion between those who, with Kant, see no circumstances in which the duty to be truthful can be abrogated, 'whatever the disadvantages accruing',[13] and those who believe deception can be justifiably undertaken at times. The absolutist view has the virtue of simplicity, but probably helps few in the area of health care. Medieval philosophers like Augustine were more concerned to distinguish between excuses that could be advanced for lies, and Aquinas went on to distinguish 'officious' lies, told with the intention of benefiting someone, from 'jocose' lies, told in fun, and from 'mischievous' lies, told in malice, which were particularly to be condemned. Both thinkers permitted concealment, and distinguished lies from statements that are, literally regarded, true, but are intended to induce false beliefs. They also introduced the 'mental reservation' controversy that lasted for centuries, but which now seems more relevant to the playground than the clinic. (What would we think of a doctor who, on being accused by a patient of having lied to him, replied that he had said what he had with his fingers crossed behind his back?) Medical thinking has always been greatly influenced by consequences, and the outcome of any line of action is a strong argument. Thus utilitarian philosophers, looking at the balance of good and evil, try to assess the degree to which a lie could increase or decrease happiness, or avoid or cause harm. But even rule utilitarians would appear to hold that a world living by 'always tell the truth' would in probability be better than a world without such a rule.[14] Most have agreed that in order for any human interaction to be valuable, it must be based on the premiss that communication will be honest. Without truthfulness, debate, discussion, even the basis of science would be pulled away. The principle of veracity seems central to the good life, and to good medicine.

Most modern thinkers in the field of medical ethics would hold that truthfulness is indeed a central principle of conduct, but that it is capable of coming into conflict with other principles, to which it must occasionally give way. On the other hand, the principle of veracity often receives support from other principles. For instance, it is hard to see how a patient can have autonomy, can make a free choice about matters concerning himself, without some measure of understanding of the facts as they influence the case; and that implies, under normal circumstances, some open, honest discussion with his advisers.[15] Equally, consent is a nonsense if it is not in some sense informed. The doctor's perspective, related to the patient's perceived needs and interests, is becoming less dominant over the patient's perspective, often expressed in terms of 'rights'. There has been a shift from the Hippocratic paternalistic view towards a view of the relationship between patient and professional as based rather on a contract or covenant. Here, at best, the patient is seen as an active or participating member of the decision-making team. Information about the patient, though not a possession in law, is seen increasingly as something to which the patient has a right of access.

The Patients' Bill of Rights is quite unequivocal.[16] This states that the patient has the right 'to informed participation in all decisions involving his health care program', a right 'to know what research and experimental protocols are being used' in the facility and what alternatives are available in the community, a right 'to a clear concise explanation of all proposed procedures in layman's terms, including the possibilities of any risk of mortality or serious side effects, problems relating to recuperation, and probability of success', and a right 'to know the identity and professional status of all those providing service'. Some professionals might be glad to know all these things too! In a strange way this approach, however laudable in itself, may come close to confusing the issue again between knowledge and truthfulness. It has by all accounts allowed the physician, on occasion, to substitute standardized data for honest communication. It certainly shows the Socratic wisdom of saying, openly, 'I do not know,' and raises the fascinating issue, seldom discussed, of how much a professional can expect or demand to be told by a patient. This has a direct bearing on whether patients have a *duty* or merely a right to be involved in decision-making—whether as a patient I can exercise my autonomy not to be autonomous. This side of the patient–professional relationship has received surprisingly little attention, and would repay further study.

Once the central position of honesty has been established, we still need to examine whether doctors and nurses really do have, as has been suggested, special exemption from being truthful because of the nature of their work, and if so under what circumstances. The analogy with the discussion of the use of force may be helpful. Few would take the absolutist view here, and most would feel that some members of society, such as the police, have at times exemption from the usual prohibition against the use of physical force. The analogy reminds us, however, that the circumstances need to be carefully examined, and there is no blanket permission. The analogy is also helpful in that we can see that there may be circumstances at either end of the scale of importance when the issues, for most people, are clear cut. In a crisis, when there is absolutely no other alternative, we condone the use of force. At the other end of the scale, there may be occasions, such as controlling a good-natured crowd, in which the use of force is accepted by all for the smooth running of society, and that the 'offence', in the sense of breaking the prohibition on the use of force against a person's will, is trivial—although the physical force required may be anything but! Similarly, there are arguments for lying at either end of the scale of importance. It may finally be decided that in a crisis there is no acceptable alternative, as when life is ebbing and truthfulness would bring certain disaster. Alternatively, the moral issue may appear so trivial as not to be worth considering (as, for example, when a doctor is called out at night by a patient who apologizes by saying, 'I hope you don't mind me calling you at this time, doctor', and the doctor replies, 'No, not at all.'). However, the force analogy alerts us to the fact that occasions of these two types are few, fewer than those in which deliberate deceit would generally be regarded as acceptable in current medical practice, and should regularly be debated 'in public' if abuses are to be avoided.[17] To this end it is necessary now to examine critically the arguments commonly used to defend lying to patients.

First comes the argument that it is enormously difficult to put across a technical subject to those with little technical knowledge and understanding, in a situation where so little is predictable. A patient has bowel cancer. With surgery it might be cured, or it might recur. Can the patient understand the effects of treatment? The symptom she is now getting might be due to cancer, there might be secondaries, and they in turn might be suppressible for a long time, or not at all. What future symptoms might occur, how long will she live, how will she die—all these are desperately important questions for the patient, but even for her doctor the answers can only be informed guesses, in an area where uncertainty is so hard to bear.

Yet to say we do not know anything is a lie. As doctors we know a great deal, and *can* make informed guesses or offer likelihoods. The whole truth may be impossible to attain, but truthfulness is not. 'I do not know' can be a major piece of honesty. To deprive the patient of honest communication because we cannot know everything is, as we have seen, not only confused thinking but immoral. Thus deprived, the patient cannot plan, he cannot choose. If choice is the crux of morality, it may also, as we have argued elsewhere, be central to health. If he cannot choose, the patient cannot ever be considered to be fully restored to health.[18]

This argument also raises another human failing—to confuse the difficult with the unimportant. Passing information to people who have more restricted background, whether through lack of experience or of understanding, can be extremely difficult and time-consuming, but this is no reason why it should be shunned. Quite the reverse. Like the difficult passages in a piece of music, these tasks should be practiced, studied, and techniques developed so that communication is efficient and effective. For the purposes of informed consent, the patient must be given the information he needs, as a reasonable person, to make a reasoned choice.

The second argument for telling lies to patients is that no patient likes hearing depressing or frightening news. That is certainly true. There must be few who do. But in other walks of life no professional would normally consider it his or her duty to suppress information simply in order to preserve happiness. No accountant, foreseeing bankruptcy in his client's affairs, would chat cheerfully about the Budget or a temporarily reassuring credit account. Yet such suppression of information occurs daily in wards or surgeries throughout the country. Is this what patients themselves want?

In order to find out, a number of studies have been conducted over the past thirty years.[19] In most studies there is a significant minority of patients, perhaps about a fifth, who, if given information, deny having been told. Sometimes this must be pure forgetfulness, sometimes it relates to the lack of skill of the informer, but sometimes with bad or unwelcome news there is an element of what is (perhaps not quite correctly) called 'denial'. The observer feels that at one level the news has been taken in, but at another its validity or reality has not been accepted. This process has been recognized as a buffer for the mind against the shock of unacceptable news, and often seems to be part of a process leading to its ultimate acceptance.[20] But once this group has been allowed for, most surveys find that, of those who have had or who could have had a diagnosis made of, say, cancer, between two-thirds and three-quarters of those questioned were either glad to have been told, or declared that they would wish to know. Indeed, surveys reveal that most *doctors* would themselves wish to be told the truth, even though (according to earlier studies at least) most of those same doctors said they would not speak openly to their patients—a curious double standard! Thus these surveys have unearthed, at least for the present, a common misunderstanding between doctors and patients, a general preference for openness among patients, and a significant but small group whose wish not to be informed must surely be respected.

We return once more to the skill needed to detect such differences in the individual case, and the need for training in such skills.

Why doctors have for so long misunderstood their patients' wishes is perhaps related to the task itself. Doctors don't want to give bad news, just as patients don't want it in abstract, but doctors have the choice of withholding the information, and in so doing protecting themselves from the pain of telling, and from the blame of being the bearer of bad news. In addition it has been suggested that doctors are particularly fearful of death and illness. Montaigne suggested that men have to think about death and be prepared to accept it, and one would think that doctors would get used to death. Yet perhaps this very familiarity has created an obsession that amounts to fear. Just as the police seem over-concerned with violence, and firemen with fire, perhaps doctors have met death in their professional training only as the enemy, never as something to come to terms with, or even as a natural force to be respected and, when the time is ripe, accepted or even welcomed.

Undeniably, doctors and nurses like helping people and derive much satisfaction from the feeling that the patient is being benefited. This basic feeling has been elevated to major status in medical practice. The principle of beneficence—to work for the patient's good—and the related principle of non-maleficence— 'first do no harm'—are usually quoted as the central guiding virtues in medicine. They are expanded in the codes, and underlie the appeal of utilitarian arguments in the context of health care. 'When you are thinking of telling a lie', Richard Cabot quotes a teacher of his as saying, 'ask yourself whether it is simply and solely for the patient's benefit that you are going to tell it. If you are sure that you are acting for his good and not for your own profit, you can go ahead with a clear conscience.'[21] But who should decide what is 'for the patient's benefit'? Why should it be the doctor? Increasingly society is uneasy with such a paternalistic style. In most other walks of life the competent individual is himself assumed to be the best judge of his own interests. Whatever may be thought of this assumption in the field of politics or law, to make one's own decisions on matters that are central to one's own life or welfare and do not directly concern others would normally be held to be a basic *right*; and hardly one to be taken away simply on the grounds of illness, whether actual or merely potential.

Thus if beneficence is assumed to be the key principle, which many now have come to doubt, it can easily ride roughshod over autonomy and natural justice. A lie denies a person the chance of participating in choices concerning his own health, including that of whether to be a 'patient' at all. Paternalism may be justifiable in the short term, and to 'kid' someone, to treat him as a child because he is ill, and perhaps dying, may be very tempting. Yet true respect for that person (adult or child) can only be shown by allowing him allowable choices, by granting him whatever control is left, as weakness gradually undermines his hold on life. If respect is important then at the very least there must be no acceptable or effective alternative to lying in a particular situation if the lie is to be justified.

Staying with the assessment of consequences, however, a third argument for lying can be advanced, namely, that truthfulness can actually do harm. 'What you don't know can't hurt you' is a phrase in common parlance (though it hardly fits with concepts of presymptomatic screening for preventable disease!) However, it is undeniable that blunt and unfeeling communication of unpleasant truths can cause acute distress, and sometimes long-term disability. The fear that professionals often have of upsetting people, of causing a scene, of making fools of themselves by letting unpleasant emotions flourish, seems to have elevated this argument beyond its natural limits. It is not unusual to find that the fear of creating harm will deter a surgical team from discussing a diagnosis gently with a patient, but not deter it from performing radical and mutilating surgery. Harm is a very personal concept. Most medical schools have, circulating in the refectory, a story about a patient who was informed that he had cancer and then leapt to his death. The intended moral for the medical student is, keep your mouth shut and do no harm. But that may not be the correct lesson to be learned from such cases (which I believe, in any case, to be less numerous than is commonly supposed). The style of telling could have been brutal, with no follow-up or support. It may have been the suggested treatment, not the basic illness, that led the patient to resort to such a desperate measure. Suicide in illness is remarkably rare, but, though tragic, could be seen as a logical response to an overwhelming challenge. No mention is usually made of suicide rates in other circumstances, or the isolation felt by ill and warded patients, or the feelings of anger uncovered when someone takes such precipitate and forbidden action against himself. What these cases do, surely, is argue, not for no telling, but for better telling, for sensitivity and care in determining how much the patient wants to know, explaining carefully in ways the patient can understand, and providing full support and 'after-care' as in other treatments.

But even if it is accepted that the short-term effect of telling the truth may sometimes be considerable psychological disturbance, in the long term the balance seems definitely to swing the other way. The effects of lying are dramatically illustrated in 'A Case of Obstructed Death?'[22] False information prevented a woman from returning to healthy living after a cancer operation, and robbed her of six months of active life. Also, the long-term effect of lies on the family and, perhaps most importantly, on society, is incalculable. If trust is gradually corroded, if the 'wells are poisoned', progress is hard. Mistrust creates lack of communication and increased fear, and this generation has seen just such a fearful myth created around cancer.[23] Just how much harm has been done by this 'demonizing' of cancer, preventing people coming to their doctors, or alternatively creating unnecessary attendances on doctors, will probably never be known.

There are doubtless many other reasons why doctors lie to their patients; but these can hardly be used to justify lies, even if we should acknowledge them in passing. Knowledge is power, and certainly doctors, though usually probably for reasons of work-load rather than anything more sinister, like to remain 'in control'. Health professionals may, like others, wish to protect themselves from confrontation, and may find it easier to coerce or manipulate than to gain permission. There may be a desire to avoid any pressure for change. And there is the constant problem of lack of time. But in any assessment, the key issues remain. Not telling the truth normally involves telling lies, and doctors and nurses have no 'carte blanche' to lie. To do so requires a justification and this justification must be strong enough to overcome the negative moral weight of the lie itself. How can we set about this assessment in practical terms?

I once was part of a coxless four making an attempt on the record for the Oxford-to-London row down the Thames. We used a vast mirror to allow the bow oarsman to steer. Most medical professionals' approach to truth-telling seems to outsiders to be back to front, reminiscent of the efforts of our boat. Better effects in truth-telling are obtained from seeing things the right way round as they really are (although I'm not sure how that could have been applied to our four!). This needs effort in several ways. It is hard, but vital, to see one's own evasion, duplicity, or equivocation for what it is: a lie. Checking whether we are telling lies is difficult, but we should not be put off making observations, any more than those ancient Greeks were put off from tasting a patient's urine for sugar. Once a lie is noticed, the Golden Rule is as good as any, 'do as you would be done by', or expressed as a negative reciprocity in the *Analects* of Confucius, 'Do not do to others what you would not want others to do to you.'[24] This requires a difficult double perspective, but is essential for making a right decision. The same principle applies to choosing the right person to whom to speak. Why tell a relative about cancer and not the patient, when the normal response is to tell only the patient? Confidentiality usually precludes us speaking to others without the patient's permission, and yet for some reason, perhaps related to crisis theory, in the discussion of cancer our usual behaviour is turned on its head. (It is hard to see such an approach going down well in other clinical situations, such as the VD clinic!). Also, if the relative is the wrong recipient, sometimes the doctor or nurse may be the wrong informer. In some circumstances it may not be the professional's duty to speak, even if he should continue to help those whose duty it clearly is, as in the case of the exhausted daughter and her elderly father quoted above (p. 188).

If the importance of open communication with the patient is accepted, we need to know when to say what. If a patient is going for investigations, it may be possible at that time, before details are known, to have a discussion about whether he would like to know the details. A minor 'contract' can be made. 'I promise to tell you what I know, if you ask me.' Once that time is past, however, it requires skill and sensitivity to assess what a patient wants to know. Allowing the time and opportunity for the patient to ask questions is the most important thing, but one must realize that the patient's apparent question may conceal the one he really wants answered. 'Do I have cancer?' may contain the more important questions 'How or when will I die?' 'Will there be pain?' The doctor will not necessarily be helping by giving an extended pathology lesson. The informer may need to know more: 'I don't want to avoid your question, and I promise to answer as truthfully as I can, but first . . .' It has been pointed out that in many cases the terminal patient will tell the doctor, not vice versa, if the right opportunities are created and the style and timing is appropriate. Then it is a question of not telling but listening to the truth.[25]

If in spite of all this there still seems to be a need to tell lies, we must be able to justify them. That the person is a child, or 'not very bright', will not do. Given the two ends of the spectrum of crisis and triviality, the vast middle range of communication requires honesty, so that autonomy and choice can be maintained. If lies are to be told, there really must be no acceptable alternative. The analogy with force may again be helpful here: perhaps using the same style of thinking as is used in the Mental Health Act, to test whether we are justified in removing someone's liberty against their will, may help us to see the gravity of what we are doing when we consider deception. It also suggests that the decision should be shared, in confidence, and be subject to debate, so that any alternative which may not initially have been seen may be considered. And it does not end there. If we break an important moral principle, that principle still retains its force, and its 'shadow' has to be acknowledged. As professionals we shall have to ensure that we follow up, that we work through the broken trust or the disillusionment that the lie will bring to the patient, just as we would follow up and work through bad news, a major operation, or a psychiatric 'sectioning'. This follow-up may also be called for in our relationship with our colleagues if there has been major disagreement about what should be done.

In summary, there are *some* circumstances in which the health professions are probably exempted from society's general requirement for truthfulness. But not telling the truth is usually the same as telling a lie, and a lie requires strong justification. Lying must be a last resort, and we should act as if we were to be called upon to defend the decision in public debate, even if our duty of confidentiality does not allow this in practice. We should always aim to respect the other important principles governing interactions with patients, especially the preservation of the patient's autonomy. When all is said and done, many arguments for individual cases of lying do not hold water. Whether or not knowing the truth is essential to the patient's health, telling the truth is essential to the health of the doctor–patient relationship.

APPENDIX
Legal and political developments, January–April 1985

MICHAEL LOCKWOOD

Since the articles in this book were prepared for publication, there have been a number of developments in Britain, especially in Parliament and the courts, that have a direct bearing on issues discussed by some of the authors. What follows is a brief summary of some of the more significant recent events. (It is, of course, inevitable that by the time the book appears, this summary will itself be at least six months out of date.)

When the Warnock Committee reported, in July 1984, the Government announced that there would be a six-month consultation period, and that they would then prepare comprehensive legislation to deal with the various issues covered by the Inquiry. In the event, however, the Government has bowed to pressure, from both inside and outside Parliament, to rush through separate legislation to outlaw the activities of commercial surrogacy agencies; according to a report in *The Times* (30 March 1985), the Government hopes to have legislation on the statute book by the summer. This was largely in response to the outcry that greeted the 'Baby Cotton' case. Mrs Kim Cotton, acting as a surrogate mother for an American couple, under the auspices of the American-owned Surrogate Parenting Agency, gave birth to a daughter on 4 January 1985. 'Baby Cotton' became the subject of a 'place of safety' order obtained by Barnet Council and was subsequently (as a result of legal action by the commissioning parents) made a ward of court. In due course the High Court ordered that the child be handed over to the commissioning couple, at which point she was flown out of the country.

Meanwhile Enoch Powell (having won fifth place in the ballot for private members' Bills) was given leave to introduce his Unborn Children (Protection) Bill, which would make it a criminal offence to have in one's possession a human embryo except for the purpose of enabling a designated woman to bear a child—a specific licence for this having to be granted by the Secretary of State for Social Services. The Bill was given a Second Reading in the Commons on 15 February 1985, by 238 votes to 66. It finally completed its Committee stage on 21 March, but only after delaying tactics by opponents of the Bill had resulted in its 'losing its place in the queue' to another private member's Bill. Since the Government has made it clear that it intends to remain 'neutral', it is overwhelmingly probable that Mr Powell's Bill will run out of time. The Government now seems likely to introduce its own package of legislation in response to the Warnock Report (on matters other than surrogacy) in the next session of Parliament. (Details are expected to be released in the summer of 1985.)

Realizing that Government-sponsored legislation on the Warnock Report was likely to be some time in coming, the Royal College of Obstetricians and Gynaecologists and the Medical Research Council (MRC) decided to organize a Voluntary Licensing Authority for doctors and other scientists engaged in human-embryo research. On 29 March 1985, Dame Mary Donaldson, who is to chair the Authority, announced that it would comprise four nominees each from the Royal College and the MRC, and four non-medical representatives, who were to be Mrs Penelope Leach, the Revd Professor G. R. Dunstan, Sir Cecil Clothier, and Miss Susan Hampshire. (See *The Times*, 30 March 1985.)

On 22 February 1985, the House of Lords handed down a decision in the case of *Sidaway* v. *Bethlem Royal Hospital and the Maudsley Hospital Health Authority and Others*, that bears on the status, in English law, of the concept of *informed consent*. (See 'Law Report', *The Times*, 22 February 1985, p. 28, and 'What should a doctor tell', *British Medical Journal*, 290 (1985), pp. 780–1.) Mrs Amy Sidaway had had an operation, in October 1974, to relieve persistent pain caused by injury to her elbow. This operation went badly wrong, resulting in partial paralysis to her left side, presumably due to damage to the spinal cord. Mrs Sidaway contended that, had she known that there was a small risk of damage to the spinal cord, she would not have agreed to the operation, and that the doctor in question had accordingly been negligent in not informing her of this risk.

The Lords (partly influenced by the fact that the doctor in the case was no longer alive, and therefore could not be brought forward as a witness) were unanimous in dismissing the plaintiff's appeal against an earlier adverse judgement. They differed, however, in their guidance on the law. Lord Diplock held that the 'Bolam test' should be held to apply in such cases. This refers to the case of *Bolam* v. *Friern Barnet Hospital Management Committee* ([1957] 1 WLR 582), in which the judge directed the jury as follows as regards the standard of care required of a doctor:

The test is the standard of the ordinary skilled man exercising and professing to have that special skill . . . It is sufficient if he exercises the ordinary skill of an ordinary competent man exercising that particular art.

The specific reference is to treatment; but Diplock held that the doctor's duty to advise and warn the patient of risks was to be judged by the same standard. (All the medical witnesses agreed that the surgeon's decision not to warn Mrs Sidaway of the risk of damage to the spinal cord and its possible consequences was in accordance with a practice accepted at the time as proper by a responsible body of opinion amongst neurosurgeons, which is the Bolam criterion.)

Lord Bridge argued along very similar lines, but added the qualification that a judge might nevertheless 'come to the conclusion that disclosure of a particular risk was so obviously necessary to an informed choice on the part of a patient that no reasonably prudent medical man would fail to make it'. In such a case, the court might overrule accepted medical opinion. Bridge cited, in illustration of the sort of risk he had in mind, a 10 per cent risk of a stroke (this example being drawn from the Canadian case of *Reibl* v. *Hughes*). Lord Templeman, without citing Bolam, was in broad agreement with Diplock and Bridge.

Lord Scarman presented a dissenting opinion. He rejected the Bolam test as determining the scope of a doctor's duty to warn his patient of possible risks attending a proposed course of treatment, on the grounds that it was inappropriate that the medical profession itself should be allowed to decide what doctors had a legal duty to tell their patients. The starting point, Scarman argued, should be the patient's right to make his own decisions. English law should, he said, recognize a duty, on the part of doctors, to warn of any *material* risks inherent in the treatment being proposed; and the test of materiality should be whether in the circumstances of the particular case the court was satisfied that a reasonable person in the patient's position would be likely to regard the risk as significant. (Professor Ian Kennedy, whose own position in these matters is closely akin to that taken by Scarman, was actually cited in Scarman's judgement.)

In a nutshell, while the other Lords applied a 'reasonable doctor' test (albeit with qualifications), Scarman argued for a 'reasonable patient' test. (See entry on 'informed consent' in the Glossary, p. 245 below.)

By the time this book appears, the Lords will probably have ruled on the Gillick Appeal. (See the Postscript to Ian Kennedy's article above, pp. 64–75.) Moreover, the Government's Bill on surrogate motherhood agencies may well have become law, and their detailed plans for legislation on the other issues covered in the Warnock Report should be known. It is perhaps worth stressing, however, that if the vote on the Second Reading of Powell's Bill is anything to go by, it will be difficult for the Government to get through, on a free vote, legislation that permits experiments on human embryos. This itself may partly account for the Government's tardiness in introducing a Bill, since the Cabinet is believed to be broadly in agreement with the recommendations of the Warnock Report.

NOTES

Chapter 1 (pp. 9–31)

1 In revising this paper for publication I have been grateful for a number of constructive criticisms, particularly those of Michael Smith, Stephen Walsh, Richard Swinburne, and Donald MacKay.

2 This point is made very clearly in an excellent article by D. M. MacKay: 'The Use of Behavioural Language to Refer to Mechanical Processes', *British Journal for the Philosophy of Science*, XIII, 50 (1962), pp. 89–103.

3 This term is originally due to David Wiggins. See his *Identity and Spatio-Temporal Continuity* (Oxford: Basil Blackwell, 1967), pp. 7, 29.

4 The idea, also exploited in one of my later examples, of using imagined future pain as a way of testing our intuitions about identity, is one I have borrowed from Bernard Williams. See his 'The Self and the Future', *Philosophical Review*, 79, No. 2 (April, 1970), pp. 161–80, reprinted in John Perry (ed.), *Personal Identity* (Berkeley: University of California Press, 1975), pp. 179–98.

5 John Locke, *Essay Concerning Human Understanding*, 2nd ed. (1694), Ch. 27, as reprinted in Perry, op. cit. (see n. 4 above), pp. 33–52.

6 Thomas Reid, 'Of Memory', in A. D. Woozley (ed.), *Essays on the Intellectual Powers of Man* (1785) (London: Macmillan, 1941). The relevant chapter, 'Of Mr. Locke's Account of Our Personal Identity', is reprinted in Perry, op. cit. (see n. 4 above), pp. 113–18.

7 Derek Parfit, 'Personal Identity', *Philosophical Review*, 80, No. 1 (January, 1971), as reprinted in Perry, op. cit. (see n. 4 above), pp. 199–223.

8 This suggestion is originally due to A. J. Ayer. See his *The Problem of Knowledge* (London: Macmillan, 1956), pp. 221–2, and also 'The Concept of a Person' in *The Concept of a Person and Other Essays* (London: Macmillan, 1963), pp. 113–14. Though he makes the suggestion, Ayer does not (to his credit) ever endorse it as an adequate analysis of personal identity.

9 Examples of this sort have been part of the philosophical folklore for

at least twenty years. A very similar example is discussed at length by Derek Parfit in his new book *Reasons and Persons* (Oxford: Oxford University Press, 1984), Part III. I recommend the discussion of personal identity in this book to anyone interested in thinking seriously about these issues: like the book in general, it is powerful and ingenious. But I am bound to say that Parfit's whole approach to the problem of personal identity seems to me, nevertheless, profoundly misguided. In particular, his insistence that psychological continuity, however caused, suffices for survival strikes me as very implausible. His argument for this relies on a supposed analogy between, on the one hand, imaginary cases such as teletransportation (my Laker example), in which psychological continuity (as between the human beings who respectively enter the 'departure' and leave the 'arrival' booths) is sustained by means other than neurophysiological continuity, and, on the other hand, the provision of a blind person with prosthetic devices that, in their effects, perfectly simulate the operation of the human eye. Parfit asks:

> Would this person be seeing . . . ? If we insist that seeing must involve the normal cause, we would answer No. But even if this person cannot see, what he has is just as good as seeing, both as a way of knowing what is within sight, and as a source of visual pleasure. If we accept the Psychological Criterion, we can make a similar claim. If psychological continuity does not have its normal cause, some may claim that it is not true psychological continuity. We can claim that, even if this is so, this kind of continuity is just as good as ordinary continuity. (*Reasons and Persons*, pp. 208–9.)

The analogy seems to me a poor one. We can, to be sure, take an instrumental view of our eyes: eyes, we may think, are things for seeing with; anything that produces the right experiences on the right occasions (and has the appropriate external appearance) is as good as nature's own issue. But is the continuity of brain structure likewise to be thought of instrumentally—as just a device for generating psychological continuity? Not if what we care about here is our survival (with or without psychological continuity). Such an instrumental view would follow only if it could be independently demonstrated that psychological continuity was the essence of survival (real essence, in Locke's terms, not merely nominal essence), or alternatively that it was in any case all that it was rational to care about. If one thinks, as I do, that the continuity of brain structure is constitutive of our continuing identity or survival, and psychological continuity is merely a manifestation of the latter, then it will matter crucially what the cause of any given instance of such continuity really is. For on that will depend the answer to the question whether what it manifests is true survival or merely a counterfeit.

10 Reports that Edwards had been experimenting on live human embryos first appeared in September 1982, in the *Daily Express* and the *Daily Star*, based on a Press Association report. The story was quickly taken up by other newspapers, including *The Times*, where it prompted a stern editorial. (See 'Embryos in the Laboratory', *The Times*, 25 September 1982.) Two days later the British Medical Association issued a warning to medically qualified doctors not to co-operate with Edwards. Edwards himself promptly denied the charge, insisting that 'At no time have I adopted any procedure in relation to a human embryo other than reimplantation or observation.' (See 'Medical fears of living organ banks', *The Times*, 29 September 1982, and 'Microscopic Life', by Oliver Gillie, *Sunday Times*, 3 October 1982.) Subsequently, Edwards sued Express Newspapers plc, publishers of both the *Daily Express* and the *Daily Star*, for libel, and on 22 June 1984 was awarded substantial damages in the High Court. (See *The Times*, 22 June 1984.) Edwards has, however, made it abundantly clear on several occasions that he would like to be allowed to experiment on live human embryos and that he does not consider it unethical to do so at a sufficiently early stage: as he says in a letter to *The Times* (6 June 1984), 'We believe that the stages soon after fertilisation are undifferentiated and that full moral protection must be conferred later, before neural tissue and sense organs enter the advanced stages.' See also 'Microscopic Life', op. cit. (see above) and 'Embryos: the case for research' by Nicholas Timmins, *The Times*, 26 June 1984, where Edwards is quoted as saying 'We must do this research . . . I believe the benefits to be gained considerably outweigh any objections to the study of early embryos . . . the need for knowledge is greater than the respect to be accorded to an early embryo.'

It is sometimes said that it is irrational to make a fuss about experimenting on human embryos (presumably painlessly) while not making a similar fuss about simply discarding such embryos, or about our present abortion law, sanctioning as it does the destruction not merely of early embryos, but also of foetuses at a much more advanced stage of development. From a purely utilitarian standpoint, this objection is obviously well taken: if embryos are going to be destroyed anyway, why not experiment on them first? But from a more Kantian perspective, it might be argued that there was a significant difference between merely discarding an embryo and actually experimenting on it. From the standpoint of someone who thinks that the embryo is a human being, the latter is, as the former is not, a violation of the principle that one should never treat a human being merely as a means but always as an end in himself. For the same reason, perhaps, the carrying out of medical experiments on prisoners, even convicted murderers, without their consent would strike many people as a worse violation of human rights than capital punishment.

11 Benjamin Libet, '"Human Life" Testimony', Letters, *Science*, 213 (1981), pp. 154–6.

12 Peter Singer and Deane Wells, *The Reproduction Revolution: New Ways of Making Babies* (Oxford: Oxford University Press, 1984), pp. 97–8.

13 The question of whether brain death and brain life are, from a moral standpoint, analogous to each other crucially depends, however, on what one takes the rationale of the brain death criterion of death to be. Jonathan Glover, for example, seems to think that this is an essentially revisionary definition of death, grounded in the consideration that the destruction of the brain structures required to sustain awareness, by making it impossible for a person ever to regain consciousness, thereby takes away a precondition for continued life having any moral value. (See his *Causing Death and Saving Lives* (Harmondsworth: Penguin Books, 1977), pp. 43–5.) But if that were the only rationale, there would clearly be no parallel, morally speaking, between the brain-dead individual and the foetus or embryo before brain development. For in due course, in the latter case, consciousness will come; in that respect the embryo or early foetus might be held to be in a position that was more closely analogous to that of a reversibly comatose patient: the physiological preconditions for awareness are lacking at present but will be there in the future. This point is made by Callahan:

> An objection to the use of a common criterion of life for both nascent embryos and dying persons might be based on one important distinction . . . with the 'death' of the brain (while the rest of the body remains 'alive') comes the loss of all potentiality for personhood; its physiological basis is irretrievably lost. In the instance of a zygote or early embryo, however—even before the advent of brain waves—the potentiality for personhood exists. (Daniel Callahan, *Abortion: Law, Choice and Morality* (New York: Macmillan, 1970), p. 389.)

The main burden of this paper is to give a different, deeper rationale for brain death, in terms of what our identity consists in, according to which the analogy between brain death and brain life is restored. If I am right about this, then the conception of brain death, properly understood, so far from being revisionary, on the contrary encapsulates the essence of what death has actually consisted in all along.

Some doctors, when they speak of 'brain death' have in mind not so much 'whole-brain death' as brain-stem death. This is sometimes defended on the grounds that, with the permanent cessation of brain-stem function, respiration and blood circulation cannot be maintained without artificial aid; such a criterion is thus continuous with the traditional criteria which would take the permanent loss of heartbeat and of breathing to mark the end of life. I cannot see that this view has anything to recommend it, philosophically speaking. For the possession of a functional brain stem, like the maintenance of heartbeat and respiration, surely have only a contingent connection with the persistence of higher brain function, which is what really counts here. This last point seems to be widely appreciated within the medical profession. One reason—perhaps the main reason—why doctors generally favour as a criterion of death the irreversible loss of function in the brain stem or, alternatively, the entire brain, as opposed to the irreversible loss of higher brain function, as might seem more logical, is the absence of any general agreement as to how the latter should be diagnosed. Patients with a flat EEG, at one time, have not infrequently been known subsequently to recover consciousness, where the brain stem was still functional; whereas irreversible loss of function in the brain stem seems invariably (though doubtless contingently) to carry with it irreversible loss of higher brain function as well. The whole issue is, in fact, extremely tangled. Those who wish to pursue it can be recommended to read Chapter 4 of Frank Harron, John W. Burnside, and Tom L. Beauchamp, *Health and Human Values* (New Haven: Yale University Press, 1983), pp. 63–84, and also 'Whole-brain death reconsidered' by Alister Browne, with a commentary by C. Pallis, *Journal of Medical Ethics*, 9, No. 1 (March 1983), pp. 28–37.

14 S. Kripke, *Naming and Necessity* (Oxford: Basil Blackwell, 1980), pp. 116–44 (original version published 1972).

15 J. L. Mackie, *Problems from Locke* (Oxford: Oxford University Press, 1976), pp. 199–203.

16 H. Putnam, 'Meaning and Reference', *Journal of Philosophy* (1973), reprinted in S. P. Schwartz (ed.), *Naming, Necessity and Natural Kinds* (Ithaca, NY: Cornell University Press, 1977) and H. Putnam, *Philosophical Papers*, Vol. 2 (Cambridge: Cambridge University Press, 1975).

17 See Parfit, op. cit. (see n. 9 above), pp. 205–8.

18 The emphasis here on neural organization, as opposed to function, means that the beginning of human life may be antecedent to the onset of awareness: the foetus may start life in a state of dreamless sleep or even coma. The brain structures whose continuity over time are, in my view, constitutive of a human being's continuing identity have in some sense to be structures that are capable of sustaining awareness. But the sense I have in mind is a fairly weak one. Consider the following question: is Karen Quinlan dead? I think this is an open question. It may well be that it is beyond the power of current or foreseeable medical science ever to restore consciousness to her, in which case there is no point in keeping her body ticking over. But that does not make her dead. Whether or not Karen Quinlan is dead is a question of whether the neural structures whose continuity over time constitutes her continuing identity as a human being have or have not been destroyed. If they have not, then she is still alive, even if there are other things wrong with her—that is, other things wrong with the 'support system' for the relevant structures—which are keeping her in a state of coma. In that case there is something that would count as waking Karen Quinlan up, whether or not we are currently able to do it—waking her up, that is, as opposed to constructing, perhaps in the same brain, a new human being. (I am told that it is actually very likely by now that the relevant brain structures have atrophied, the relevant cells died, in which case Karen Quinlan is already dead, according to my criterion.) That may help to make it clear in what sense, precisely, the structures I appeal to have to be 'capable' of sustaining awareness.

19 The evidence relevant to this point is surveyed by Clifford Grobstein, *From Chance to Purpose* (Reading, Mass.: Addison-Wesley, 1981, Ch. V.), drawing heavily on an article by Tryphena Humphrey ('Function of the Nervous System During Pre-natal Life', in U. Stave (ed.), *Prenatal Physiology* (New York: Plenum, 1978), pp. 651–83). The situation (to judge from these sources) is roughly as follows. At six weeks there is a rudimentary nervous system, but no nervous activity; neurotransmitter substances are absent. At from seven to eight weeks the first reflexes appear—only spinal reflexes, however, in the first instance. Then from nine to ten weeks after conception, the first non-reflex, spontaneous movements are observed. It is just possible that these first spontaneous movements are a manifestation of sentience, even though the balance of evidence is against it. (Such movements are superficially not unlike those observed in tadpoles, or even creatures that lack a nervous system, such as protozoa.) On the available evidence, and assuming that sentience requires nervous

activity in the brain, Grobstein concludes that sentience may be confidently ruled out only during the first eight weeks of development, but probably does not appear until a month or so later. According to Tryphena Humphrey, behaviour observed before eighteen weeks almost certainly involves only the lower brain, the mesencephalon and the brain stem, and the spinal cord, as opposed to the diencephalon and the telencephalon, which independent evidence would suggest are alone responsible for awareness.

One interesting point that emerges from Tryphena Humphrey's article concerns the apparent thumb-sucking in some foetuses, photographs of which have been exploited to good effect by anti-abortion groups. Humphrey points out that such behaviour has, in reality, nothing interestingly in common with genuine infantile thumb-sucking—in particular, that no *sucking* or even puckering of the lips is, in these cases, taking place at all.

20 I was somewhat taken aback to discover, since writing this paper, that what I am calling the 'brain life' conception of when human life begins has, for nearly twenty years, had a wide currency amongst Catholic writers. Thus, Rudolph Ehrensing, in 'When Is It Really Abortion?', *The National Catholic Reporter* (25 May 1966) writes (p. 4) that the presence of a 'human person' requires 'the existence of a living human brain in some form' and insists that 'it is not the potential for structuring matter in the form of a body, a human brain, that calls for the presence of a human person, but the actual accomplishment, the actual in-corporation of matter'. He adds: 'If the developing embryo is not yet a human person, then under some circumstances the welfare of actually existing persons might supersede the welfare of the developing human tissue.' Similar views are expressed by Roy U. Schenk ('Let's Think About Abortion', *The Catholic World*, 207 (April 1968), p. 16), Wilfried Ruff, S. J. ('Das embryonale Werden des Menschen', *Stimmen der Zeit*, 181 (1968), pp. 331–55 and 'Personalitat im embryonalen Werden', *Theologie und Philosophie*, 45 (1970), pp. 24–59), and Bernard Haring, who, in a book bearing the imprimatur of the Roman Catholic Bishop of Northampton, writes: 'it does seem that the theory which presents hominization as dependent on the development of the cerebral cortex has some probability' (Bernard Haring, *Medical Ethics* (Middlegreen: St Paul Publications, 1974), p. 84). It should be stressed, however, that Haring does not take this line of thought to legitimize abortion: 'the mere theory of hominization as dependent on the development of the cerebral cortex does not provide any ground for depriving the embryo of the basic human right to life'. This last remark, however,

seems to pay more heed to orthodoxy than to logic: why should the embryo be thought to possess 'the basic human right to life' if it is not yet a human being?

21 See 'British Medical Association working group on in vitro fertilisation and embryo replacement and transfer, Interim report on human in vitro fertilisation and embryo replacement and transfer', *British Medical Journal*, 286 (14 May 1983), pp. 1594–5, reprinted in Singer and Wells, op. cit. (see n. 12 above), pp. 227–33.

22 Judith Jarvis Thomson, 'A Defense of Abortion', *Philosophy and Public Affairs*, 1 (1971), pp. 47–66, reprinted in Tom L. Beauchamp (ed.), *Ethics and Public Policy* (Englewood Cliffs, NJ: Prentice-Hall, 1975), pp. 319–21.

23 For the distinction between what Hare calls the 'intuitive' and 'critical' levels of moral thinking, see the Glossary (p. 245 below) and also his *Moral Thinking* (Oxford: Oxford University Press, 1981), Ch. 22, pp. 25–43.

24 The reader may be puzzled that I here say ten weeks, when in note 19 I cite scientific opinion as definitively ruling out sentience only in the first eight weeks. Actually, there is no inconsistency. In the context of pregnancy, 'ten weeks' means ten weeks menstrual age, calculated, that is, from the beginning of the last cycle, i.e. menstruation. Since ovulation takes place in the middle of the menstrual cycle, and conception usually within twelve hours afterwards, ten weeks, in this sense, means approximately eight weeks from conception. The following explanation is from a standard medical textbook:

> A pregnant woman usually will see her obstetrician when two successive menstrual bleedings have failed to occur. By that time her recollection about the coitus is usually vague and it is readily understandable that the day of fertilization is difficult to determine.
>
> The obstetrician calculates the date of birth as 280 days or 40 weeks from the first day of the last menstrual bleeding. This day is usually remembered quite accurately. In women with regular 28-day menstrual periods, the method is rather accurate, but when the cycles are irregular substantial miscalculations may be made. It must be remembered that the time between ovulation and the succeeding menstrual bleeding is constant (14 days ± 1 day), but the time between ovulation and the preceding menses is highly variable. (Jan Langman, *Medical Embryology*, 3rd ed. (Baltimore: Williams and Wilkins, 1975), pp. 86–7.)

25 Clearly, also, one should set an earlier time limit for any abortion of a normal child, where the mother's life or physical health is not

endangered by continued pregnancy, than applies at present, since babies have now been born alive a full five weeks before the present limit on abortions. It is morally indefensible, in my view, for a doctor to abort a healthy foetus that is capable of being born alive; and unreasonable of the mother to request that this be done. The present time limit could be retained, however, for abortions that were genuinely therapeutic, or proposed because of some grave and inoperable defect in the foetus, such that it was judged better, if not for the child itself then at least for those on whom the burden of caring for it would fall, that it not be allowed to live. Steps should also be taken to ensure that no foetus ever suffers in the course of an abortion: there is disturbing evidence that at present some do.

26 Michael Tooley, 'Abortion and Infanticide', *Philosophy and Public Affairs*, 2 (1972), pp. 37–65.

27 Peter Singer, 'Killing Humans and Killing Animals', *Inquiry*, 22 (1979), pp. 145–56.

28 Michael Lockwood, 'Singer on Killing and the Preference for Life', *Inquiry*, 22 (1979), pp. 157–70.

29 The references to Singer, Tooley, and Glover are to the works cited above (notes 27, 26, and 13 respectively). Hare's views on these matters are to be found in his 'Abortion and the Golden Rule', *Philosophy and Public Affairs*, 4 (1975) and 'The Abnormal Child: Moral Dilemmas of Doctors and Parents', *Documentation in Medical Ethics*, 3, reprinted as 'Survival of the Weakest' in S. Gorovitz (ed.), *Moral Problems in Medicine* (Engelwood Cliffs, NJ: Prentice-Hall, 1976), pp. 364–9, where he says (p. 369) 'I do not think that the harm you are doing to the foetus or the unsuccessfully operated upon newborn infant by killing them is greater than that which you are doing to Andrew by stopping him from being conceived and born.'

30 Glover, op. cit. (see n. 13 above), pp. 159–63.

Chapter 2 (pp. 32–75)

1 President's Commission for the Study of Ethical and Legal Problems in Medicine and Biomedical and Behavioral Research, *Making Health Care Decisions* (Washington: US Government Printing Office, 1982).

2 Ibid., p. 170.

3 Ibid., pp. 171–2.

4 [1984] 1 All ER 365.

5 Ibid.

6 Ibid., p. 370.

7 Ibid., p. 373.

8 Ibid., p. 375.

9 Ibid., p. 374.

10 G. Williams, *Textbook of Criminal Law*, 2nd ed. (London: Stevens, 1982), p. 338.

11 J. C. Smith and Brian Hogan, *Criminal Law*, 4th ed. (London: Butterworths, 1978).

12 Ibid., p. 114.

13 Op. cit. (see n. 10 above), p. 331.

14 [1975] 2 All ER 684, 686.

15 [1975] AC 653.

16 Ibid., 698.

17 [1959] 1 QB 11.

18 Ibid., 20.

19 *R.* v. *Meyrick*, (1929) 21 Cr. App. Rep. 94, 102.

20 See n. 16 above.

21 See n. 4 above.

22 Op. cit. (see n. 4 above), p. 371.

23 Ibid., p. 372.

24 [1976] 2 QB 217.

25 Op. cit. (see n. 4 above), p. 372.

26 [1984] 1 All ER 277.

27 [1960] 1 QB 129.

28 Op. cit. (see n. 11 above), p. 124.

29 Op. cit. (see n. 26 above), p. 285.

30 Op. cit. (see n. 27 above).

31 Professor Williams captures the problem with two propositions which are opposing and each of which is circular: 'The law compels the performance of this duty; therefore doing it cannot be a crime. To do this would be a crime; therefore doing it cannot be a legal duty.' Op. cit. (see n. 10 above), p. 344.

32 Op. cit. (see n. 4 above), p. 371.

33 Op. cit. (see n. 10 above), p. 346.

34 Ibid., p. 334.

Chapter 3 (pp. 76–91)

1 The report of the working party referred to is to be published by Oxford University Press under the title *The Ethics of Clinical Research on Children*. The Chairman was Professor Gordon Dunstan. The philosophical chapter in it was drafted by me and revised by the working party. I used my draft as the basis of a paper given at the 7th International Congress of Logic, Methodology and Philosophy of Science at Salzburg in July 1983, which will appear in the *Proceedings* of the Congress. It was also given in Oxford as a companion lecture to that here published; and this explains why I have not in this lecture entered into very full theoretical discussion of the issue between utilitarians and deontologists. My general utilitarian position is set out and defended in my recent book *Moral Thinking* (Oxford: Oxford University Press, 1981), where references will also be found to papers of mine on other relevant topics, including justice. Another paper, 'Arguing about Rights' is in *Emory Law Journal*, 33 (1984). The report of the working party gives references to the cases cited and other useful bibliographical information.

2 This trial is reported in J. T. Lanman, L. P. Guy, and J. Dancis, 'Retrolental fibroplasia and oxygen therapy', *Journal of the American Medical Association*, 155 (1954), pp. 223–6. There is also an excellent recent book on the subject, which goes into the history; it is William A. Silverman, *Retrolental Fibroplasia: A Modern Parable* (New York: Grunne and Stratton, 1980). This trial was controversial at the time. Silverman points out that there are methodological doubts surrounding it which have never been satisfactorily resolved.

3 See Michael Lockwood, 'Controls or victims: the ethics of non-treatment in clinical trials', *Oxford Medical School Gazette*, XXXI, No. 1 (Trinity Term 1979), pp. 29–31. An expanded version of the article is published under the title 'Sins of Omission? The Ethics of Non-Treatment in Clinical Trials' in *Proceedings of the Aristotelian Society*, Supp. Vol. LVII (1983), pp. 207–22.

4 See references in n. 1 above.

5 Stuart Hampshire, 'Morality and Pessimism', the 1972 Leslie Stephen Lecture, reprinted in Stuart Hampshire (ed.), *Public and Private Morality* (Cambridge: Cambridge University Press, 1978), pp. 1–22.

6 The review system proposed in Florida is described by D. B. Wexler, 'Behavior Control and Other Behavior Change Procedures', *Criminal Law Bulletin*, 11 (1975), also incorporated in his *Mental Health Law: Major Issues* (New York: Plenum, 1981).

7 See letter from Professor Ian Kennedy, *The Times*, 11 February 1982, p. 17.

Chapter 4 (pp. 92–110)

1 Thomas S. Szasz, 'Involuntary Mental Hospitalization: A Crime Against Humanity', in Tom L. Beauchamp and L. Walters (eds), *Contemporary Issues in Bioethics* (Encino, Ca.: Wadsworth, 1978), pp. 551–7.

2 E. N. Clark and I. Grey, 'The Diogenes syndrome', *Lancet*, 1975, pp. 366–8.

3 See G. K. Wilcock, J. A. M. Gray, and P. M. M. Pritchard, *Geriatric Problems in General Practice* (Oxford: Oxford University Press, 1982).

4 Tom L. Beauchamp and James F. Childress, *Principles of Biomedical Ethics* (New York and Oxford: Oxford University Press, 1979), pp. 67–70.

5 G. J. Alexander, P. H. D. Lewin, R. M. Alderman, L. Wisenfelder, and D. Meiklejohn, *The Aged and the Need for Surrogate Management* (Syracuse, NY: Syracuse University Press, 1972).

6 Parliamentary Debates, Commons, *Hansard*, 444 (1948), Column 1623.

7 *Report of the Committee on Homosexual Offences and Prostitution* (London: HMSO, 1957).

8 Patrick Devlin, 'The Enforcement of Morals', *Proceedings of the British Academy*, 45 (1959), reprinted as 'Morals and the Criminal Law' in *The Enforcement of Morals* (Oxford: Oxford University Press, 1965), pp. 1–25.

9 H. L. A. Hart, *Law, Liberty and Morality* (Oxford: Oxford University Press, 1963).

10 Keith Thomas, *Religion and the Decline of Magic* (London: Weidenfeld and Nicolson, 1971).

11 Ibid., p. 760.

12 Ibid., p. 672.

13 Ibid., p. 673.

14 K. V. Thomas, 'Anthropology and the Study of English Witchcraft', in Mary Douglas (ed.), *Witchcraft Confessions and Accusations* (London: Tavistock Publications, 1970), p. 67.

15 J. S. Mill, *On Liberty* (1859), ed. Gertrude Himmelfarb (Harmondsworth: Penguin Books, 1974), p. 68.

16 A. A. Baker, 'Slow euthanasia or—"she will be better off in hospital"',
   British Medical Journal, 1976, 2, pp. 571–7.

17 M. A. Lieberman, V. N. Prock, and S. S. Tobin, 'Psychological
   Effects of Institutionalisation', *Journal of Gerontology*, 23 (1968),
   pp. 343–53.

Chapter 5 (pp. 111–25)

1 See, for example, Brian O'Shaughnessy, *The Will: A Dual Aspect
   Theory*, 2 vols (Cambridge: Cambridge University Press, 1980).

2 This point is stressed by A. C. MacIntyre who, having 'define[d] free
   behaviour as rational behaviour', says that 'behaviour is rational—in
   this arbitrarily defined sense—if, and only if, it can be influenced or
   inhibited by the adducing of logically relevant considerations'. He
   adds: 'it is important to see that to define free behaviour as rational
   behaviour, as I have done, does not lead to the paradox that a free act
   is never a foolish act. To say that a man's behaviour is open to
   alteration by logically relevant considerations is not to say that he
   alters his behaviour in actual fact.' (A. C. MacIntyre, 'Determinism',
   Mind, LXVI (1957), pp. 28–41.) It was Michael Lockwood who first
   acquainted me with this conception of autonomy and who brought
   MacIntyre's article to my attention.

3 J. Benson, 'Who Is the Autonomous Man?', *Philosophy*, 58, No. 223
   (January 1983), pp. 5–7.

4 J. S. Mill, *On Liberty* (1859), ed. Gertrude Himmelfarb (Harmondsworth: Penguin Books, 1974), p. 69.

5 Cf. I. Kant, *Groundwork of the Metaphysics of Morals*, tr. H. J. Paton
   (New York: Harper and Row, 1964), p. 80. I shall not give further
   detailed references. A useful summary of Kant's work is given in Paul
   Edwards (ed.), *The Encyclopaedia of Philosophy* (New York and London:
   Collier-Macmillan, 1972) in W. H. Walsh's entry on Kant.

6 See Hare's remarks on freedom and freedom of speech in his *Moral
   Thinking* (Oxford: Oxford University Press, 1981), p. 167 and pp.
   155 f., respectively, and also his 'What is Wrong with Slavery',
   Philosophy and Public Affairs, 8, No. 2 (Winter 1979), pp. 103–21.

7 Op. cit. (see n. 4 above), p. 68.

8 J. Gray, *Mill on Liberty: A Defence* (London: Routledge and Kegan
   Paul, 1983).

9 Op. cit. (see n. 4 above), p. 70.

10 Someone might object that it was always an empirical possibility
   that happiness would not be maximized, on any given occasion, by

respect for autonomy. I think the utilitarian reply (following Hare) would be that it is indeed a possibility, but that unless we have very good empirical evidence that it is a strong probability, we should act as though the far stronger probability (that welfare or happiness would be maximized by respecting autonomy) were true. Hare adds that prudent utilitarians will tend to discount low probabilities in favour of high probabilities in doing the calculations and will tend to discount cases in which self-interest may be the real motive in favour of cases where self-interest can be ruled out. But for the deontologist pluralist it remains an objection to utilitarianism that even in theory respect for autonomy might be overridden as a general principle if the empirical evidence showed a high probability that doing so would maximize welfare. See Hare, *Moral Thinking*, op. cit. (see n. 6 above), and John Gray, 'Indirect Utility and Fundamental Rights', in Ellen Frankel Paul and Fred D. Miller (eds), *Human Rights* (Oxford and New York: Basil Blackwell, 1984), pp. 73–91.

11 Op. cit. (see n. 4 above), p. 68.

12 Sophisticated definitions and analyses of paternalism abound in the (mostly American) very considerable literature. A useful selection appears in Gorovitz *et al.* (eds), *Moral Problems in Medicine* (Englewood Cliffs, NJ: Prentice-Hall, 1976). C. M. Culver and D. Gert also analyse these issues in their *Philosophy and Medicine: Conceptual and Ethical Issues in Medicine and Psychiatry* (New York and Oxford: Oxford University Press, 1982).

13 E. Kubler-Ross, *On Death and Dying* (London: Tavistock Publications, 1970), p. 32.

14 A. Shaw, 'Dilemmas of "informed consent" in children', *New England Journal of Medicine*, 289, No. 17 (1973), pp. 885–90.

15 A. Buchanan, 'Medical Paternalism', *Philosophy and Public Affairs*, 7, No. 4 (Summer 1978), as reprinted in Marshall Cohen, Thomas Nagel, and Thomas Scanlon (eds), *Medicine and Moral Philosophy* (Princeton, NJ: Princeton University Press, 1981), pp. 214–34.

16 Ibid., p. 224.

17 Ibid., p. 227.

18 Such a theory is put forward by Hare in his 'Ethical Theory and Utilitarianism', in H. D. Lewis (ed.), *Contemporary Moral Philosophy 4* (London: Allen and Unwin, 1976) and is developed in detail in his *Moral Thinking*, op. cit. (see n. 6 above).

19 R. Bayliss, 'A health hazard', *British Medical Journal*, 285 (1982), pp. 1824–5.

20 M. D. Kirby, 'Informed consent: what does it mean?', *Journal of Medical Ethics*, 9, No. 2 (June 1983), pp. 69–75.

21 E. D. Pellegrino, 'Toward a reconstruction of medical morality: the primacy of the act of profession and the fact of illness', *Journal of Medicine and Philosophy*, 4, No. 1 (1979), pp. 32–56.

22 Cf. M. S. Komrad, 'A defence of medical paternalism: maximising patients' autonomy', *Journal of Medical Ethics*, 9, No. 1 (March 1983), pp. 38–44, and R. Sherlock, 'Consent, competency and ECT: some critical suggestions', *Journal of Medical Ethics*, 9, No. 3 (September 1983), pp. 141–3.

23 Anonymous (Editorial), 'Impaired autonomy and rejection of treatment', *Journal of Medical Ethics*, 9, No. 3 (September 1983), p. 132.

24 An interesting interdisciplinary discussion of this cluster of issues is to be found in R. Sherlock, H. Lesser, and P. J. Taylor, 'Competent but irrational refusal of ECT—must it be accepted?', *Journal of Medical Ethics*, 9, No. 3 (September 1983), pp. 141–51.

Chapter 6 (pp. 126–37)

1 This is traditionally called the Sorites. An important discussion of some basic issues is Michael Dummett, 'Wang's Paradox', *Synthese*, 30 (1975), reprinted in his *Truth and Other Enigmas* (London: Duckworth, 1978), pp. 248–68. (Wang's paradox is an inverted version of the Sorites.)

2 I am alluding here to the theory of virtue which Aristotle advances in his *Nicomachean Ethics*. Aristotle's doctrine is that every virtue of character lies between two vices or failings which represent extremes in opposite directions. Thus courage, for example, is viewed by Aristotle as a mean between the deficiency that is cowardice and the excess we call rashness.

3 Nelson Goodman, *Languages of Art—An Approach to a Theory of Symbols* (Indianapolis: Hackett Publishing Co., 1976), pp. 110–11.

4 The conventional Prisoners' Dilemma picture of the arms race overlooks the respects in which it is a co-operative undertaking. (See entry on Prisoners' Dilemma in the Glossary, p. 247 below.)

5 Michael Tooley is an example. See his 'Abortion and Infanticide', *Philosophy and Public Affairs*, 2 (1972), pp. 37–65, and also his new book *Abortion and Infanticide* (Oxford: Oxford University Press, 1983). I discuss this point at greater length in *Ethics and the Limits of Philosophy* (London: Fontana and Harvard University Press, 1985).

Chapter 7 (pp. 138–54)

1 This talk was given in November 1983, some seven months before the Committee of Inquiry into Human Fertilisation and Embryology presented its Report. Some things that I say here (albeit as personal opinions only) could be seen as anticipating specific recommendations of the Report; while certain other issues that are raised here are explored in the Report in greater depth. Where appropriate, therefore, I have given, in the Notes, references to the relevant chapters or paragraphs of the Report. (This, incidentally, is how I shall refer to it; the full title is Department of Health and Social Security, *Report of the Committee of Inquiry into Human Fertilisation and Embryology* (London: HMSO, 1984).

2 Zoe, the first child to develop successfully from a frozen embryo, was born by caesarian section in Australia on 28 March 1984, at the Queen Victoria Medical Centre of Melbourne's Monash University. It was announced at the same time that five other women who had been treated at the Centre were carrying babies that had developed from frozen embryos. One of these, a boy, was born on August 16; this was the third frozen embryo baby, a second having been born in Rotterdam in July. On 16 July 1984, Edwards and Steptoe announced that they also had two patients whose pregnancies were due to the implantation of embryos that had been frozen and subsequently thawed. One of these was born on 8 March 1985.

In June 1984, it was revealed that the Queen Victoria Medical Centre was facing a bizarre ethical dilemma concerning what have come to be known as the 'orphan embryos'. A California couple who were treated for infertility at the Centre, had been killed in a plane crash leaving in storage at the Centre two frozen embryos, which it had been planned to introduce into the wife's uterus at a later date. This raises such questions as (a) whether the embryos should be implanted in the womb of some other woman, assuming that one could be found who wished to have this done, or whether it would be all right to use the embryos for research purposes or simply to discard them; and (b) whether, assuming that they were successfully implanted, the resulting children should be regarded as eligible to inherit the very considerable fortune left by the couple. A further twist was added to the story by the subsequent revelation that the embryos had as their genetic father, not the husband, but an un-identified Australian. On 9 September 1984 the Waller Committee, set up in 1982 by the Victoria State Government to investigate essentially the same range of issues as my own committee, presented its Report, which recommended that frozen embryos should be removed from storage if their parents had died without leaving explicit instructions. The State Government said it would allow three months for public debate before introducing any legislation implementing the Waller Committee's recommendations. The latest news (reported in *The Times*, 24 October 1984)) is, however, that the upper house of the Victoria State Parliament has passed a special amendment to allow the 'orphan embryos' to be adopted and implanted—this after a campaign on their behalf led by Mrs Margaret Tighe, President of the Right to Life Organisation of Victoria. It is reported that over ninety women have volunteered to give the embryos a womb and a home. The whole issue may well turn out to have been academic: Professor Carl Wood, who heads the *in vitro* fertilization team at the Centre, has expressed the opinion that, in view of the fact that the embryos were frozen in June 1981, before the improvements in technique that made possible the birth of Zoe, it is actually rather unlikely, in this particular case, that the embryos could be successfully implanted. (See 'Orphan Embryos', *Nature*, 309 (28 June 1984), p. 738.) Nevertheless, the case is a dramatic illustration of the sort of problems, legal and ethical, that the new techniques raise.

There are two recommendations in the Report that bear on this sort of case (which was envisaged by the Committee). First, we recommend, at 10.12, that if both members of a couple who have stored an embryo die, 'the right to use or dispose of any embryo stored by that couple should . . . pass to the storage authority'. (If one dies, we recommend that the right should pass to the surviving member.) Secondly, we 'recommend that legislation should be introduced to provide that any child born following IVF, using an embryo that had been frozen and stored, who was not *in utero* at the date of the death of the father shall be disregarded for the purposes of succession to and inheritance from the latter'.

3 A case that has attracted considerable publicity recently concerns that of a woman in France, whose husband had contracted cancer of the testicles, and who, having been warned that the chemotherapy might leave him sterile, had deposited some of his semen with a sperm bank, apparently intending that the woman who later became his wife should be inseminated with it if it turned out to be impossible for them to have children by normal means. In the event, the man died of the cancer a mere two days after their wedding. The widow then asked the sperm bank to hand over to her the frozen sperm, so that she could have a child by her dead husband. When they refused, she sued the sperm bank to have the semen released. (A legal

complication was that, under a Napoleonic law, a child born to a woman more than 300 days after her husband's death is to be considered illegitimate.) In August 1984 a French court ruled in the woman's favour, saying however that they did not wish their ruling to be taken as a precedent. The woman was subsequently inseminated, but failed to conceive. (See *The Times*, 11 July and 2 August 1984 and 11 January 1985.)

This situation is, in effect, anticipated in the Report. Thus, we remark, in 10.7, that 'a man might wish to store semen before undergoing surgery, chemotherapy or radiotherapy that is likely to make him sterile . . . , in the hope that he may father a child by artificial insemination at a later date'. And we say, in 4.4, that 'we have grave misgivings about AIH in one type of situation. A man who has placed semen in a semen bank may die and his widow may then seek to be inseminated . . . This may give rise to profound psychological problems for the child and the mother.' Finally, at 10.10, we say 'The use by a widow of her dead husband's semen for AIH is a practice which we feel should be actively discouraged. Despite our own views on the matter . . . , we realise that such requests may occasionally be made.'

4 The issues raised by the freezing and storage of human sperm, eggs, and embryos are discussed in Chapter 10 of the Report.

5 This technique is known as 'embryonic biopsy'; see the Report, 12.12–12.13.

6 Cf. Report, 5.1–5.9.

7 Home Office and Scottish Department, *Report of the Departmental Committee on Human Artificial Insemination* (Chairman: the Earl of Feversham) (London: HMSO, 1960).

8 R. Snowden and G. D. Mitchell, *The Artificial Family* (London: George Allen and Unwin, 1981).

9 R. Snowden, G. D. Mitchell, and E. M. Mitchell, *Artificial Reproduction: A Social Investigation* (London: George Allen and Unwin, 1983). Referring to my committee's Report, Snowden and Mitchell have said in a recent letter to *The Times* (9 August 1984) that they 'are broadly in agreement with its recommendations, particularly as they apply to artificial insemination . . . '

10 This has been recommended by the Law Commission; my committee endorsed their recommendations: see the Report, 4.17.

11 The Report specifically recommends that, where the husband has consented to AID, the law should be changed to permit him to be entered on the birth certificate as the father; see 4.25. We also

expressed the belief that there should be greater openness about AID; an increase in provision, which we should welcome, may help to make AID more acceptable. But clearly, a change in attitudes towards male infertility is also required, if the present pretence and deception is to be rendered unnecessary. See the Report, 4.27–4.28.

12 There have been several such cases already. A recent case, which received considerable publicity, concerned a woman in New South Wales in Australia, who had agreed to act as a surrogate for a professional couple in Sydney. 'I thought I would be a good candidate', the woman was reported as saying. 'I enjoy being pregnant and having babies. With six kids I thought I had enough responsibility. But I just don't want to give this baby up.' The child's natural father, describing his and his wife's acute disappointment— they had already made extensive preparations and had even bought nappies—said the situation was 'a disaster, an absolute disaster. It's hit my wife harder than me.' As chance would have it, the New South Wales Artificial Conception Act, under which the natural father, in this sort of case, is denied any claim to paternity, had come into force the day before the mother's refusal to give the child up. (See *The Times*, 3 August 1984.)

13 The question of surrogacy is dealt with in Chapter 8 of the Report. It is also the subject of a minority Expression of Dissent, pp. 87–9.

14 Cf. Report, 2.3–2.4.

15 The legislation that has in fact been recommended by the Committee would make it a criminal offence not only to advertise a surrogacy service but also for a doctor, or any other third party, to arrange a surrogate pregnancy; it would not, however, make criminals of the couple involved, nor of the surrogate mother herself, who would still, under the legislation we have proposed, be able to make a private surrogacy arrangement, albeit one that was unenforceable in law. See the Report, 8.18–8.19.

16 Such was the view of a minority of the Committee in regard to the legislation we in fact proposed; see the Expression of Dissent referred to in n. 13 above.

17 The setting up of such infertility centres is recommended in the Report, at 2.15.

18 Such, in essence, were the conclusions of a ten-year study carried out under the joint aegis of the SSRC and the DHSS. Nicola Madge summarizes the position thus:

> The fulfilment of emotional needs is . . . crucial to a child's well-being and development. It remains undisputed that children need

to form attachments during infancy if there are not to be severe emotional repercussions, and that they need to have a fairly stable caretaker on whom to depend during childhood. Generally natural parents provide this emotional support, although it may be given by foster or adoptive parents, by a member of staff in an institutional setting, or by someone else with whom an intimate and long-standing relationship is established. It is not necessary . . . for infants to receive the almost undivided attention of their mothers, even during the first few years of life . . . What is important, however, is that children feel emotionally secure and experience good relationships within the family.

This is from 'An Introduction to Families at Risk', in Nicola Madge (ed.), *Families at Risk* (SSRC/DHSS Studies in Deprivation and Disadvantage, 8) (London: Heinemann, 1983), p. 4. See also M. Rutter, *Maternal Deprivation Reassessed*, 2nd ed. (Harmondsworth: Penguin Books, 1981).

19 Sex selection is discussed at length in the Report, though we felt unable to make any positive recommendations, save that the matter be kept under review. See the Report, 9.4–9.12.

20 My committee did not wish to encourage this practice and was therefore opposed to providing prospective parents seeking sperm donors with descriptions of donors sufficiently detailed to make it possible. See the Report, 4.19–4.21.

21 Patrick Devlin, 'The Enforcement of Morals', *Proceedings of the British Academy*, 45 (1959), reprinted under the title 'Morals and the Criminal Law' in Patrick Devlin, *The Enforcement of Morals* (Oxford: Oxford University Press, 1965), pp. 1–25.

22 *Report of the Committee on Homosexual Offences and Prostitution* (London: HMSO, 1957). It is worth noting that, although the view on the relationship between society's morals and the law that I have here been expressing has something in common with Devlin's, there is in fact a close analogy between the approach of my committee to the issue of surrogacy and that of Lord Wolfenden's Committee to the issue of prostitution. Just as Wolfenden's Committee did not wish the mere act of prostitution to be a crime, so we did not wish the practice of surrogacy itself to be a crime either. Our recommended ban on the activities of third parties in arranging surrogacy is analogous to the Wolfenden Report's recommendation that the activities of pimps should continue to be outlawed. I hasten to add, however, that I am not in the least suggesting that surrogacy is to be equated, morally speaking, with prostitution.

23 R. M. Dworkin, 'Lord Devlin and the Enforcement of Morals', in Richard A. Wassertrom (ed.), *Morality and the Law* (Belmont, Ca.: Wadsworth, 1971), pp. 55–72.

Chapter 8 (pp. 155–86)

1 The official title of the Warnock Report is Department of Health and Social Security, *Report of the Committee of Inquiry into Human Fertilisation and Embryology* (Chairman: Dame Mary Warnock DBE), Cmnd. 9314 (London: HMSO, 1984). References to the Report will, unless otherwise indicated, be to paragraphs, rather than to pages.

2 On 'Face the Press', Channel 4, 22 July 1984.

3 Thomas Nagel, 'Death', in *Mortal Questions* (Cambridge: Cambridge University Press, 1979), p. 10.

4 *Abortion and the Right to Life: A joint statement of the Catholic Archbishops of Great Britain* (Abbots Langley, Herts.: Catholic Information Services, 1980), para. 12.

5 Warnock Report, 11.17.

6 Ibid., Expression of Dissent: B. Use of Human Embryos in Research, pp. 90–3.

7 Ibid., Foreword, pp. 2–3.

8 Ibid., 11.22.

9 Remarks to the effect that minds are indivisible are to be found in many places in Leibniz's writings, e.g. in *A New System of the Nature and the Communication of Substances* (1695), paras. 4 and 11, in L. E. Loemaker (ed.), *G. W. Leibniz: Philosophical Papers and Letters*, 2nd ed. (Dordrecht, 1969), pp. 454 and 456.

10 René Descartes, *Meditations on First Philosophy*, 2nd ed. (1642), reprinted in Elizabeth Anscombe and Peter Thomas Geach (eds), *Descartes, Philosophical Writings* (London: Nelson, 1964), Sixth Meditation, p. 121. Kant criticizes Descartes's argument in his *Critique of Pure Reason*, 2nd ed., 416n. There is an excellent discussion of this issue in Jonathan Bennett, *Kant's Dialectic* (Cambridge: Cambridge University Press, 1974), pp. 85–7.

11 See R. W. Sperry, 'Hemisphere Deconnection and Unity in Conscious Awareness', in *American Psychologist*, XIII (1968), pp. 723–33. Further references may be found in Thomas Nagel's 'Brain Bisection and the Unity of Consciousness', in his *Mortal Questions*, op. cit. (see n. 3 above), pp. 146–64.

12 For philosophical discussion of the implications of these experiments, see the article by Thomas Nagel referred to in n. 11 above and also Derek Parfit, *Reasons and Persons* (Oxford: Oxford University Press, 1984), pp. 244–66. Parfit assumes that Sperry's interpretation is correct; Nagel questions it, and suggests that the unity of consciousness may not be an all-or-nothing affair. Nagel thinks that the experimental evidence that Sperry cites is to some extent counteracted by the fact that, in most normal circumstances, the behaviour of 'split-brain' subjects seems perfectly integrated. This is indeed a striking fact; it is one that has caused some workers in the field to speculate that the two hemispheres of the brain may be associated with distinct streams of consciousness even in normal people! From this point of view, the reason why the two hemispheres co-operate so well, even when the corpus callosum is severed, is that they have had a lifetime of practice. That speculation aside, I should have thought that the behavioural integration was sufficiently explained (a) by the fact that the two hemispheres are receiving consistent, if not identical, information and (b) by the fact that the two hemispheres are highly motivated towards co-operation. It is interesting, in connection with the latter point, that Donald and Valerie MacKay found recently that they were quite unable, with 'split-brain' subjects, to get the two hemispheres to compete against each other in a simple game: each hemisphere would constantly try to help the other (D. M. and Valerie MacKay, 'Explicit dialogue between left and right half-systems of split brains', *Nature*, 295 (1982), pp. 690–1. Finally, even in normal circumstances, there are sometimes dramatic (and rather eerie) instances, in 'split-brain' subjects, of dissociation. One I have already mentioned (that of the wife and the husband's hands); in another case a woman complained that she would decide which dress she wanted to wear, but when she went to the wardrobe, her left hand would reach out and take a different one.

13 See Warnock Report, Expression of Dissent: C. Use of Human Embryos in Research, p. 94, and also 11.25–11.30.

14 Warnock Report, 11.18.

15 Ibid., 11.20.

16 Council for Science and Society, *Human Procreation: ethical aspects of the new techniques*, Report of a Working Party (Oxford: Oxford University Press, 1984), pp. 53–4.

17 A poll carried out recently by MORI for the Order of Christian Unity showed that 34 per cent of people interviewed would be in favour of allowing experiments on human embryos to continue up to

the point at which the embryo was capable of feeling pain. Seeing that just over 50 per cent wanted a complete ban on such experiments, and there was presumably a fair number of 'don't knows', this suggests that a substantial majority of those who were in favour of allowing such experiments at all would approve of a six week cut-off point. (See Andrew Veitch, 'Human embryo research "should be forbidden"', *Guardian*, 28 September 1984, p. 6, col. 1.) But no doubt some would argue that, given that public opinion is divided, one ought to compromise between this and a total ban by choosing some earlier time limit. It appears to have been on some such basis as this that the Council for Science and Society Working Party ended up recommending a fourteen-day time limit, just like the Warnock Committee. See *Human Procreation*, op. cit. (see n. 16 above), p. 82.

18 The likely impact on human-embryo research of passing into law the Warnock Committee's recommendations is assessed in a recent article by Omar Sattaur, 'New conception threatened by old morality', *New Scientist*, 103, No. 1423 (27 September 1984), pp. 12–17. The therapeutic possibilities are briefly surveyed in Robert Edwards and Patrick Steptoe, *A Matter of Life* (London: Sphere Books, 1981), pp. 213–15.

19 Warnock Report, 11.17.

20 See John Harris, 'In Vitro Fertilization: The Ethical Issues I', *Philosophical Quarterly*, 33 (1983), p. 224.

21 Mary Warnock, 'In Vitro Fertilization: The Ethical Issues II', *Philosophical Quarterly*, 33 (1983), pp. 241–2.

22 Warnock Report, Foreword, p. 2.

23 See Warnock, op. cit. (see n. 21 above), pp. 244–5 and Ted Honderich, 'On Liberty and Morality-Dependent Harms', *Political Studies*, 30 (1982).

24 See Lord Justice Patrick Devlin, 'The Enforcement of Morals', *Proceedings of the British Academy*, 45 (1959), reprinted as 'Morals and the Criminal Law' in *The Enforcement of Morals* (Oxford: Oxford University Press, 1965) and in Richard A. Wassertrom (ed.), *Morality and the Law* (Belmont, Ca.: Wadsworth, 1971), pp. 24–48.

25 By a 'secondary principle', Mill means a principle more specific and of more limited scope than the principle of utility itself, the justification of which is that adherence to it may generally be expected to promote utility, and that it is easier to apply than the principle of utility itself. See John Stuart Mill, *Utilitarianism*, in James M. Smith and Ernest Sosa (eds), *Mill's Utilitarianism* (Belmont, Ca.: Wadsworth, 1969), pp. 51–3.

26 *Report of the Committee on Homosexual Offences and Prostitution* (Chairman: Sir John Wolfenden), Cmnd. 247 (London: HMSO, 1957).

27 Home Office, *Report of the Committee on Obscenity and Film Censorship* (Chairman: Bernard Williams), Cmnd. 7772 (London: HMSO, 1979).

28 Ibid., Ch. 5.

29 Ibid., pp. 51–2.

30 Devlin, op. cit. (see n. 24 above).

31 Warnock Report, Foreword, p. 2; see also 11.20.

32 Warnock, op. cit. (see n. 21 above), p. 245.

33 Ibid., pp. 245–7.

34 Warnock Report, 11.24.

35 John Stuart Mill argues this in his *On Liberty* (1859).

36 Warnock, op. cit. (see n. 21 above), p. 245.

37 This phrase is borrowed from John Rawls, see *A Theory Of Justice* (Oxford: Oxford University Press, 1973), p. 12.

38 Warnock Report, 8.17; see also Expression of Dissent: A. Surrogacy, p. 87.

39 There has been a test case that is reported in *Human Procreation*, op. cit. (see n. 16 above), p. 68:

> In re C (a minor) (1978) a professional man and the woman with whom he was living were unable to have children. They found a prostitute who was willing to bear the man's child by AID for £3000. When the child was born the prostitute refused to give it up. The couple, who were married by now, could not persuade the woman to hand over the child, despite offering additional inducements of a car and, in desperation, their house. The father brought wardship proceedings unsuccessfully and the court refused to recognize the validity of the contract, declaring it to be pernicious and against public policy, and describing the father and his wife as 'most selfish and irresponsible'.

40 Warnock Report, 8.19.

41 Ibid., Expression of Dissent: A. Surrogacy, pp. 87–9.

42 Ibid., 8.18.

43 Bill Handel, a Californian lawyer who runs the agency, made this claim on the 'Today' programme, BBC Radio 4, 24 September 1984.

44 Mary Warnock said this in the course of an interview on the 'Today' programme (see n. 43 above).

45 See Peter Singer and Deane Wells, *The Reproduction Revolution: New Ways of Making Babies* (Oxford: Oxford University Press, 1984), pp. 79–80.

46 Warnock Report, 8.10 (see also 4.10).

47 Keith Ward has been reported as saying that surrogacy 'could change the family quite radically', clearly meaning by 'change' change for the worse. (See the *Daily Express*, 24 September 1984, p. 1, col. 4).

48 Warnock Report, Foreword, p. 2.

49 See Stuart Hampshire, 'Morality and Pessimism', in Stuart Hampshire (ed.), *Public and Private Morality* (Cambridge: Cambridge University Press, 1978), pp. 1–22 and Warnock Report, p. 3.

50 The quotation from Anna McCurley is from the *Daily Mirror*, p. 1, col. 1, that from Peter Bruinvels from the *Daily Star*, p. 5, col. 3, and that from Nicholas Winterton from the *Daily Express*, p. 2, col. 5, all 24 September 1984.

51 See the *Daily Star*, p. 4, col. 1, 24 September 1984.

52 Hampshire, op. cit. (see n. 49 above), p. 11.

53 Ibid., pp. 12–13.

54 Warnock, op. cit. (see n. 21 above), p. 246. The quotation from Hume comes from the *Treatise*, Book III, Part I, Section 2.

55 The theory was originally put forward in R. M. Hare, 'Ethical Theory and Utilitarianism', in H. D. Lewis (ed.), *Contemporary Moral Philosophy 4* (London: Allen and Unwin, 1976); it is developed in greater detail in his *Moral Thinking* (Oxford: Oxford University Press, 1981).

56 Warnock, op. cit. (see n. 21 above), pp. 247–8.

57 Hampshire, op. cit. (see n. 49 above), p. 10.

58 Warnock, op. cit. (see n. 21 above), p. 247.

59 H. L. A. Hart, 'Immorality and Treason', *The Listener* (30 July 1959), pp. 162–3, reprinted in Wassertrom (ed.), op. cit. (see n. 24 above), p. 54.

60 Ronald Dworkin, 'Lord Devlin and the Enforcement of Morals', in Wassertrom (ed.), op. cit. (see n. 24 above), p. 69.

61 Hart, op. cit. (see n. 59 above), p. 54.

62 Devlin, op. cit. (see n. 24 above), p. 38.

63 See Edmund Burke, 'Speech to the Electors of Bristol (1774)', in *The Works of the Right Honourable Edmund Burke*, Vol. II (London: Oxford University Press, 1906), pp. 164–5.

64 In a Harris opinion poll commissioned recently by the *Observer*, 56 per cent of those polled agreed with the statement 'Homosexuals should have the same rights as heterosexuals', with only 27 per cent disagreeing. (See Katherine Whitehorn, 'Britons Observed, Part 2: Morals, Tolerance and Religion', *Observer Magazine*, 23 September 1984, p. 58.

65 Warnock Report, 8.17.

66 In the same MORI opinion poll referred to in n. 17 above, over 57 per cent of those asked were, however, found to be opposed to that form of surrogacy involving IVF, in which the bearing mother is not the genetic mother; only 31 per cent approved of this technique.

Chapter 9 (pp. 187–202)

1 *Primum non nocere*—this is a latinization of a statement which is not directly Hippocratic, but may be derived from the *Epidemics* Book 1 Chapter II: 'As to diseases, make a habit of two things—to help, or at least do no harm.' *Hippocrates*, 4 Vols. (London: William Heinemann, 1923–31), Vol. I. Translation W. H. S. Jones.

2 Cases collected by the author in his own practice.

3 Case collected by the author.

4 Quoted in Reiser, Dyck, and Curran (eds), *Ethics in Medicine, Historical Perspectives and Contemporary Concerns* (Cambridge, Mass.: MIT Press, 1977).

5 American Medical Association, 'Text of the American Medical Association New Principles of Medical Ethics' *American Medical News* (August 1–8 1980), 9.

6 To be found in Reiser *et al.*, op. cit. (see n. 4 above).

7 Lawrence Henderson, 'Physician and Patient as a Social System', *New England Journal of Medicine*, 212 (1935).

8 Quoted in W. H. Auden and Louis Kronenberger (eds), *The Faber Book of Aphorisms* (London: Faber, 1962).

9 The uncertainty principle is a consequence of quantum mechanics discovered by Heisenberg in 1927.

10 Sissela Bok, *Lying: Moral Choice in Public and Private Life* (London: Quartet, 1980).

11 R. S. Downie and Elizabeth Telfer, *Caring and Curing: A philosophy of medicine and social work* (London: Methuen, 1980).

12 For a summary of these ideas, see Sissela Bok, 'Truth-telling II' in Warren T. Reich (ed.), *Encyclopaedia of Bioethics* (New York: Free Press, 1978).

13 Immanuel Kant, 'On a Supposed Right to Lie from Benevolent Motives', translated by T. K. Abbott, in Kant's *Critique of Practical Reason and other works on the Theory of Ethics* (London: Longmans, 1909).

14 Discussed in Robert Veatch, *A Theory of Medical Ethics* (New York: Basic Books, 1981).

15 Alastair Campbell and Roger Higgs, *In That Case* (London: Darton, Longman and Todd, 1982).

16 George J. Annas, *The Rights of Hospital Patients: The Basic ACLU Guide to a Hospital Patient's Rights* (New York: Avon Books, 1976).

17 John Rawls, *A Theory of Justice* (Cambridge, Mass.: Harvard University Press, Belknap Press, 1971).

18 Op. cit. (see n. 15 above).

19 Summarized well in Robert Veatch, 'Truth-telling I' in *Encyclopaedia of Bioethics*, op. cit. (see n. 12 above).

20 The five stages of reacting to bad news, or news of dying, are described in *On Death and Dying* by Elizabeth Kubler-Ross (London: Tavistock, 1970). Not everyone agrees with her model. For another view see a very stimulating article 'Therapeutic Uses of Truth' by Michael Simpson in E. Wilkes (ed.), *The Dying Patient* (Lancaster: MTP Press, 1982). 'In my model there are only two stages—the stage when you believe in the Kubler-Ross five and the stage when you do not.'

21 Quoted in Richard Cabot, 'The Use of Truth and Falsehood in Medicine; an experimental study', *American Magazine* Vol. 5 (1903) pp. 344–9.

22 Roger Higgs, 'Truth at the last—A Case of Obstructed Death?', *Journal of Medical Ethics*, 8 (1982), 48–50, and Roger Higgs, 'Obstructed Death Revisited', *Journal of Medical Ethics*, 8 (1982), pp. 154–6.

23 Susan Sontag, *Illness as Metaphor* (New York: Farrar, Straus and Giroux, 1978).

24 Quoted in Bok, op. cit. (see n. 10 above), p. 93n.

25 Cicely Saunders, 'Telling Patients', *District Nursing* (now *Queens Nursing Journal*) (September 1963), pp. 149–50, 154.

FURTHER READING

General

Norman Autton, *Doctors Talking* (London and Oxford: Mowbray, 1984).

Tom L. Beauchamp and James F. Childress, *Principles of Biomedical Ethics* (New York and Oxford: Oxford University Press, 1979).

Charles M. Culver and Bernard Gert, *Philosophy in Medicine* (New York and Oxford: Oxford University Press, 1982).

Frank Harron, John Burnside, and Tom Beauchamp, *Health and Human Values* (New Haven and London: Yale University Press, 1983).

Ian Kennedy, *The Unmasking of Medicine*, paperback ed. (London: Granada, 1983).

Chapter 1: When does a life begin?

Jonathan Glover, *Causing Death and Saving Lives* (Harmondsworth: Penguin Books, 1977), especially Chs 9–11.

Clifford Grobstein, *From Chance to Purpose* (Reading, Mass.: Addison-Wesley, 1981), especially Ch. V.

Michael Lockwood, 'Singer on Killing and the Preference for Life', *Inquiry*, 22 (1979), pp. 157–70.

John Mackie, *Problems from Locke* (Oxford: Oxford University Press, 1976), Ch. 6.

Derek Parfit, *Reasons and Persons* (Oxford: Oxford University Press, 1984), Part III.

John Perry (ed.), *Personal Identity* (Berkeley: University of California Press, 1975).

Peter Singer, 'Killing Humans and Killing Animals', *Inquiry*, 22 (1979), pp. 145–56.

Peter Singer and Deane Wells, *The Reproduction Revolution* (Oxford: Oxford University Press, 1984), pp. 84–98.

Judith Jarvis Thomson, 'A Defense of Abortion', *Philosophy and Public Affairs*, 1 (1971), pp. 47–66, reprinted in Tom L. Beauchamp (ed.), *Ethics and Public Policy* (Englewood Cliffs, NJ: Prentice-Hall, 1975), pp. 319–21.

Michael Tooley, 'Abortion and Infanticide', *Philosophy and Public Affairs*, 2 (1972), pp. 37–65.

Michael Tooley, *Abortion and Infanticide* (Oxford: Oxford University Press, 1983).

Chapter 2: The doctor, the pill, and the fifteen-year-old girl

Tom L. Beauchamp and James F. Childress, *Principles of Biomedical Ethics* (New York and Oxford: Oxford University Press, 1979), Chs 3, 7, and 8.

Bernard Dickens, 'The Modern Function and Limits of Parental Rights', 97, *Law Quarterly Review* 462 (1981).

J. Eekelaar, 'What are Parental Rights?', 89, *Law Quarterly Review* 210 (1973).

Gillick v. West Norfolk and Wisbech Area Health Authority, [1984] 1 All ER 365.

Law Reform Commission of Canada, *Consent to Medical Care* (Ottawa: LRCC, 1980).

Neil MacCormick, 'Children's Rights: a Test-Case for Theories of Right', in *Legal Right and Social Democracy: Essays in Legal and Political Philosophy* (Oxford: Oxford University Press, 1982), pp. 159–66.

President's Commission for the Study of Ethical and Legal Problems in Medicine and Biomedical and Behavioral Research, *Making Health care Decisions* (Washington: US Government Printing Office, 1982).

Robert Veatch, *A Theory of Medical Ethics* (New York: Basic Books, 1981), especially Chs 6, 7, and 8.

Glanville Williams, *Textbook of Criminal Law* (London: Stevens, 1979), especially Chs 8 and 13.

Chapter 3: Little human guinea-pigs

A. G. M. Campbell, 'Infants, Children and Informed Consent', based on inaugural lecture given at the University of Aberdeen, *British Medical Journal*, 1974, 3, pp. 334–8.

G. Dworkin, 'Legality of consent to nontherapeutic medical research on infants and young children', *Archives of Disease in Childhood*, 53 (1978), pp. 443–6.

Raanan Gillon, 'Clinical research on children' (unsigned editorial), *Journal of Medical Ethics*, 8 (1982), pp. 3–4.

R. M. Hare, 'Arguing About Rights', *Emory Law Journal*, forthcoming.

R. M. Hare, *Moral Thinking* (Oxford: Oxford University Press, 1981).

R. M. Hare, 'The Ethics of Clinical Experimentation on Children', *Proceedings of the 7th International Congress of Logic, Methodology and Philosophy of Science*, forthcoming.

J. T. Lanman, L. P. Guy, and J. Dancis, 'Retrolental fibroplasia and oxygen therapy', *Journal of the American Medical Association*, 155 (1954), pp. 223–6.

Michael Lockwood, 'Sins of Omission? The Ethics of Non-Treatment in Clinical Trials', *Proceedings of the Aristotelian Society*, Supp. Vol. LVII (1983), pp. 207–22.

Richard A. McCormick, SJ, 'Proxy Consent in the Experimentation Situation', *Perspectives in Biology and Medicine*, Autumn 1974.

M. H. Pappworth, *Human Guinea Pigs: Experimentation in Man* (London: Routledge and Kegan Paul, 1967).

A. H. Schwartz, 'Children's concepts of research hospitalisation', *New England Journal of Medicine*, 287 (1972), pp. 589–92.

William A. Silverman, *Retrolental Fibroplasia: A Modern Parable* (New York: Grune and Stratton, 1980).

Society for the Study of Medical Ethics, *The Ethics of Clinical Research on Children* (Oxford: Oxford University Press, 1985).

Working party on ethics of research in children, 'Guidelines to aid ethical committees considering research involving children', *British Medical Journal*, 280 (1980), pp. 229–31.

Chapter 4: The ethics of compulsory removal

G. J. Alexander, T. H. D. Lewin, R. M. Alderman, L. Wisenfelder, and D. Meiklejohn, *The Aged and the Need for Surrogate Management* (Syracuse, NY: Syracuse University Press, 1972).

A. A. Baker, 'Slow euthanasia or—"she will be better off in hospital"', *British Medical Journal*, 1976, 2, pp. 571–7.

E. Clark and I. Grey, 'The Diogenes syndrome', *Lancet* (1975), pp. 366–8.

J. A. Muir Gray, 'Section 47', *Journal of Medical Ethics*, 7 (1981), pp. 146–9.

Reports of the Commissioners, *Report of the Royal Commission on the Poor Laws and Relief of Distress* (1905–1909), Part IV, especially Chs 6 and 7.

Keith Thomas, 'Anthropology and the Study of English Witchcraft', in Mary Douglas (ed.), *Witchcraft Confessions and Accusations* (London: Tavistock Publications, 1970).

Keith Thomas, *Religion and the Decline of Magic* (London: Weidenfeld and Nicolson, 1971).

S. Webb and B. Webb, *The Minority Report of the Poor Law Commission* (London: Longman Green, 1909).

G. K. Wilcock, J. A. M. Gray, and P. M. M. Pritchard, *Geriatric Problems in General Practice* (Oxford: Oxford University Press, 1982).

Chapter 5: Autonomy and consent

J. Benson, 'Who Is the Autonomous Man?', *Philosophy*, 58 (1983), pp. 5–17.

A. Buchanan, 'Medical Paternalism', *Philosophy and Public Affairs*, 7, No. 4 (Summer 1978), reprinted in Marshall Cohen, Thomas Nagel, and Thomas Scanlon (eds), *Medicine and Moral Philosophy* (Princeton, NJ: Princeton University Press, 1981), pp. 214–34.

Howard Brody, 'Autonomy revisited', *Journal of the Royal Society of Medicine*, forthcoming.

Charles M. Culver and Bernard Gert, *Philosophy in Medicine* (New York and Oxford: Oxford University Press, 1982), Chs 3, 7, and 8.

C. M. Culver, R. B. Ferrell, and R. M. Green, 'ECT and special problems of informed consent', *American Journal of Psychiatry*, 137 (1980), pp. 586–97.

R. Gillon, 'Impaired autonomy and rejection of treatment' (unsigned editorial), *Journal of Medical Ethics*, 9, No. 3 (September 1983), pp. 131–2.

J. Gray, *Mill on Liberty: A Defence* (London: Routledge and Kegan Paul, 1983).

I. Kant, *Groundwork of the Metaphysics of Morals*, tr. H. J. Paton (New York: Harper and Row, 1964).

M. D. Kirby, 'Informed consent: what does it mean?', *Journal of Medical Ethics*, 9, No. 2 (June 1983), pp. 69–75.

M. S. Komrad, 'A defence of medical paternalism: maximising patients' autonomy', *Journal of Medical Ethics*, 9, No. 1 (March 1983), pp. 38–44.

A. C. MacIntyre, 'Determinism', *Mind*, LXVI (1957), pp. 28–41.

J. S. Mill, *On Liberty* (1859), ed. Gertrude Himmelfarb (Harmondsworth: Penguin Books, 1974).

Onora O'Neill, 'Paternalism and partial autonomy', *Journal of Medical Ethics*, 10, No. 4 (December 1984), pp. 173–8.

E. D. Pellegrino, 'Towards a reconstruction of medical morality: the primacy of the act of profession and the fact of illness', *Journal of Medicine and Philosophy*, 4, No. 1 (1979), pp. 32–56.

A. Shaw, 'Dilemmas of "informed consent" in children', *New England Journal of Medicine*, 289 (1973), No. 17, pp. 885–90.

R. Sherlock, H. Lesser, and P. J. Taylor, 'Competent but irrational refusal of ECT—must it be accepted?', *Journal of Medical Ethics*, 9, No. 3 (September 1983), pp. 141–51.

Chapter 6: Which slopes are slippery?

Tom L. Beauchamp, 'A Reply to Rachels on Active and Passive

Euthanasia', in Tom L. Beauchamp and Seymour Perlin (eds), *Ethical Issues in Death and Dying* (Englewood Cliffs, NJ: Prentice-Hall, 1978), reprinted in part in Frank Harron, John Burnside, and Tom Beauchamp, *Health and Human Values* (New Haven and London: Yale University Press, 1982), pp. 58–61.

Tom L. Beauchamp and James F. Childress, *Principles of Biomedical Ethics* (New York and Oxford: Oxford University Press, 1979), pp. 110–13.

Michael Dummett, 'Wang's Paradox', *Synthese*, 30 (1975), reprinted in his *Truth and Other Enigmas* (London: Duckworth, 1978), pp. 248–68.

Jonathan Glover, *Causing Death and Saving Lives* (Harmondsworth: Penguin Books, 1977), pp. 164–7, 263–4.

S. Gorovitz, 'Progeny, Progress and Primrose Paths', in his *Doctors' Dilemmas: Moral Conflict and Medical Care* (New York and London: Macmillan Publishing Co. and Collier-Macmillan, 1982), pp. 164–78, reprinted in part in S. Gorovitz *et al.*, *Moral Problems in Medicine*, 2nd ed. (Englewood Cliffs, NJ: Prentice-Hall, 1983), pp. 355–63.

Germaine Grisez and Joseph Boyle, *Life and Death with Liberty and Justice: A Contribution to the Euthanasia Debate* (Notre Dame and London: Notre Dame University Press, 1979), pp. 172–4.

Bernard Williams, *Ethics and the Limits of Philosophy* (London: Fontana and Harvard University Press, 1985).

Chapter 7: The artificial family and
Chapter 8: The Warnock Report

Council for Science and Society Report, *Human Procreation: Ethical Aspects of the New Techniques* (Oxford: Oxford University Press, 1984).

Department of Health and Social Security, Scottish Home and Health Department, Welsh Office, *The Use of Fetuses and Fetal Material for Research: Report of the Advisory Group*, Chairman: Sir John Peel (London: HMSO, 1972).

Department of Health and Social Security, *Report of the Committee of Inquiry into Human Fertilisation and Embryology*, Chairman: Dame Mary Warnock (London: HMSO, 1984).

Lord Patrick Devlin, 'The Enforcement of Morals', *Proceedings of the British Academy*, 45 (1959), reprinted as 'Morals and the Criminal Law' in his *The Enforcement of Morals* (Oxford: Oxford University Press, 1965), pp. 1–25 and in Wassertrom (below), pp. 24–48.

R. M. Dworkin, 'Lord Devlin and the Enforcement of Morals', in Wassertrom (below), pp. 55–72.

Robert Edwards and Patrick Steptoe, *A Matter of Life* (London: Sphere Books, 1981).

R. G. Edwards and J. Purdy, *Human Conception In Vitro* (London: Academic Press, 1982).

Raanan Gillon, '*In vitro* fertilisation' (unsigned editorial), *Journal of Medical Ethics*, 9, No. 4 (December 1983), pp. 187–8, 199.

John Harris and Mary Warnock, '*In Vitro* Fertilization: The Ethical Issues', *Philosophical Quarterly*, 33 (1983), pp. 217–49.

H. L. A. Hart, 'Immorality and Treason', *Listener*, 30 July 1959, pp. 162–3, reprinted in Wassertrom (below), pp. 49–54.

H. L. A. Hart, *Law, Liberty and Morality* (London: Oxford University Press, 1963).

Teresa Iglesias, '*In vitro* fertilisation: the major issues', *Journal of Medical Ethics*, 10, No. 1 (March 1984), pp. 32–7.

Ian Kennedy, 'Let the law take on the test-tube', *The Times*, 26 May 1984, p. 6.

C. B. Kerr, Negative and positive eugenics II: new concepts of human quality control', in H. Messel (ed.), *The Biological Manipulation of Life* (Oxford: Pergamon Press, 1981).

J. S. Mill, *On Liberty* (1859), ed. Gertrude Himmelfarb (Harmondsworth: Penguin Books, 1974).

Home Office, *Report of the Committee on Homosexual Offences and Prostitution*, Chairman: Lord Wolfenden (London: HMSO, 1957).

Home Office, *Report of the Committee on Obscenity and Film Censorship*, Chairman: Bernard Williams (London: HMSO, 1979), Part 2, especially Ch. 5.

Home Office and Scottish Department, *Report of the Departmental Committee on Human Artificial Insemination*, Chairman: the Earl of Feversham (London: HMSO, 1960).

Omar Sattaur, 'New conception threatened by old morality', *New Scientist*, 27 September 1984, pp. 12–17.

B. F. Scarlett, Peter Singer, and Helga Kuhse, 'Debate: The moral status of Embryos', *Journal of Medical Ethics*, 10, No. 2 (June 1984), pp. 79–81.

Peter Singer and Deane Wells, *The Reproduction Revolution: New Ways of Making Babies* (Oxford: Oxford University Press, 1984).

Peter Singer, Deane Wells, and G. D. Mitchell, 'Symposium: *In vitro* fertilisation: the major issues', *Journal of Medical Ethics*, 9, No. 4 (December 1983), pp. 192–9.

Peter Singer and Bill Walters (eds), *Test-Tube Babies* (Melbourne and Oxford: Oxford University Press, 1982).

R. Snowden and G. D. Mitchell, *The Artificial Family* (London: George Allen and Unwin, 1983).

R. Snowden, G. D. Mitchell, and E. M. Mitchell, *Artificial Reproduction: A Social Investigation* (London: George Allen and Unwin, 1983).

Richard A. Wassertrom (ed.), *Morality and the Law* (Belmont, Ca.: Wadsworth, 1971).

Chapter 9: On telling patients the truth

Sissela Bok, *Lying: Moral Choice in Public and Private Life* (London: Quartet, 1980).

Sissela Bok, 'Truth-telling II', in Warren T. Reich (ed.), *Encyclopaedia of Bioethics* (New York: Free Press, 1978).

Richard Cabot, 'The Use of Truth and Falsehood in Medicine; an experimental study', *American Magazine*, 5 (1903), pp. 344–9.

Alastair Campbell and Roger Higgs, *In That Case* (London: Darton, Longman and Todd, 1982).

R. S. Downie and Elizabeth Telfer, *Caring and Curing: A philosophy of medicine and social work* (London: Methuen, 1980), especially pp. 59–66.

Raanan Gillon, 'On telling dying patients the truth' (unsigned editorial), Journal of Medical Ethics, 8, No. 3 (September 1982), pp. 115–16.

Lawrence Goldie, 'The ethics of telling the patient', *Journal of Medical Ethics*, 8, No. 3 (September 1982), pp. 128–33.

Lawrence Henderson, 'Physician and Patient as a Social System', *New England Journal of Medicine*, 212 (1955).

Roger Higgs, 'Truth at the last—a case of obstructed death', *Journal of Medical Ethics*, 8 (1982), pp. 48–50.

Roger Higgs, 'Obstructed death revisited', *Journal of Medical Ethics*, 8 (1982), pp. 154–6.

Immanuel Kant, 'On a Supposed Right to Lie from Benevolent Motives', tr. T. K. Abbott, in *Kant's Critique of Practical Reason and other works on the Theory of Ethics* (London: Longmans, 1909).

Elizabeth Kubler-Ross, *On Death and Dying* (London: Tavistock Publications, 1970).

Cicely Saunders, 'Telling Patients', *District Nursing* (now *Queens Nursing Journal*), September 1963.

Michael Simpson, 'Therapeutic Uses of Truth', in E. Wilkes (ed.), *The Dying Patient* (Lancaster: MTP Press, 1982).

Robert Veatch, 'Truth-telling I', in Warren T. Reich (ed.), *Encyclopaedia of Bioethics* (New York: Free Press, 1978).

GLOSSARY OF LEGAL, MEDICAL, AND PHILOSOPHICAL TERMS

acute   A disease is said to be acute when it is attended with symptoms of some severity and comes speedily to a crisis. Contrast **chronic**.

AID   Artificial insemination by donor, i.e. with sperm taken from someone other than the woman's husband (or male partner).

AIH   Artificial insemination by husband (used, for example, when the husband has difficulty in ejaculating during intercourse, or has a very low sperm count, and his wife is therefore artificially inseminated with semen from the husband that has been concentrated in the laboratory).

analytical   As in *analytical philosophy* or the *analytical method*, pertaining to the approach to problems (in philosophy, say, or law) that places great emphasis on a logical dissection or *analysis* of the relevant concepts.

autonomy   The capacity to make one's own decisions, usually in a way that pays proper heed to consequences and is open to reason.

autonomy, principle of   The moral principle according to which one should respect people's autonomy; that is, allow them to make their own decisions. This is to be contrasted with **paternalism**.

brain death   Irreversible loss of brain function. Usually this is taken to mean irreversible loss of function in the *brain stem*. But sometimes people speak of *whole brain death*, where what is meant is irreversible loss of function throughout the brain. As a contingent matter, irreversible loss of brain stem function seems invariably to carry with it irreversible loss of function in the midbrain and the cerebral hemispheres.

capacity   The power to give (legally or morally) valid consent to something.

chemotherapy   Treatment of malignant disease (cancer) with powerful cytotoxic (cell-killing) drugs and/or chemicals. Side-effects commonly include hair-loss and anaemia.

chromosomes   Strands of **DNA** in the cell nucleus on which the genes are located.

chronic   A chronic disease is one of long duration. Contrast **acute**.

clinical trial   A procedure whereby one or more differing forms of treatment are given to patients, usually selectively, and often by random allocation, with the aim of testing their effectiveness, or relative effectiveness.

cloning   (a) A method of fertilizing an ovum in which the chromosomes are removed and replaced by chromosomes taken from an ordinary cell. The ovum will then, in theory, develop into an organism that is genetically identical to that from which the chromosomes were taken. This has been achieved in amphibians, but not yet in human beings and probably (though this is a matter of some dispute) not in any mammal.

(b) Any method whereby a number of replicas of some biological entity are produced. Thus, one may speak of cloning DNA.

coma   A state of unconsciousness from which the subject cannot be aroused.

competence   A person's **capacity** to make valid decisions in some particular area of his or her life. A person may be competent to make decisions in one field, but not in another.

consequentialist   Applied to that form of reasoning in morals which judges the rightness or wrongness of proposed courses of action on the basis of the goodness or badness of their likely or possible outcomes (where 'outcome' may be understood to include the occurrence of the action itself). *Consequentialism* is the theory that this is ultimately the sole criterion of right and wrong. Contrast **deontological**.

corpus callosum   The tissue that links the two **hemispheres** of the brain.

curariforms   A group of powerful muscle-paralysing chemicals, mainly used to achieve muscle relaxation for the purposes of surgery. Based on the South American Indian plant-derived poison *curare*.

dementia   A state in which there is a severe impairment of normal mental functions, such as memory, thought, powers of recognition, and so forth—as in *senile dementia*, dementia associated with age.

deontological   Applied to that form of moral theory or of moral reasoning which assesses the rightness or wrongness of actions not, or not merely, on the basis of their likely or possible consequences, but on the basis of their intrinsic character, as according with or running contrary to, some specific duty, such as the duty to keep one's promises, or to tell the truth, or to respect the rights of others. (From *deon*, in Greek, meaning duty.) Contrast **consequentialist**.

diabetes   *Diabetes mellitus* (literally, 'honey fountain') is a condition in which the body cannot properly metabolize sugar, owing to a deficiency of insulin, produced by the pancreas. Treatment is by daily insulin injection and careful diet.

differentiation The process, in embryonic development, whereby different cells begin to take on different roles and characters associated with different organs and types of tissue. In the very early embryo the cells are essentially identical or *undifferentiated*; differentiation produces liver cells, nerve cells, blood cells, and so forth.

DNA Deoxyribonucleic acid—a chain molecule which, in the form of the celebrated *double helix*, makes up the **chromosomes** in the nucleus of an organism, and embodies all the genetic information.

Down's syndrome An abnormal genetic make-up resulting from a duplication of one **chromosome** (frequently chromosome 21—hence its other name of Trisomy–21). The extra chromosome is responsible for the typical facial features and often subnormal intelligence of the Down's or 'mongol' child.

EEG Electroencephalogram. This is a device that monitors electrical activity ('brain-waves') within the cerebral **hemispheres**.

electro-convulsive therapy (ECT) A treatment for depression which involves passing a mild electric current through the brain. This causes convulsions, which nowadays are controlled by a combination of restraining straps or clamps and muscle relaxants. No one has yet satisfactorily explained why this treatment should work (assuming that it does, which some might question).

embryo The word for an animal, in the early stages of its development within the womb or the egg. In the case of human beings, it is customary, in Britain, to speak of an embryo during the first six weeks of development and subsequently, until birth, of a **foetus**.

epistemology The study of knowledge, especially from an abstract, philosophical perspective.

foetus The word for an animal, in the later stages of its development in the womb or the egg. In Britain, the foetal stage in human beings is normally held to extend from six weeks after conception until birth.

gene therapy A hypothetical method of treating genetically caused disorders by replacing some or all of the defective genes in the affected subject by non-defective ones.

General Medical Council (GMC) This is the principal regulatory and disciplinary body of the British medical profession.

haemophilia A genetic blood disorder causing excessive bleeding and failure to clot after injury. The disease is inherited in a sex-linked manner, so that, although females *carry* the disease, its symptoms are usually only manifested in males.

hemispheres (of the brain) The left and right halves of the *cerebrum* or higher brain, which is associated with higher mental functions such as thought, perception, and (in human beings) language.

Hippocratic oath Ancient oath, setting out a moral framework for the profession of medicine. Attributed to the ancient Greek physician, Hippocrates of Cos (*c.* 460–*c.* 380 BC), but more probably derived from the Pythagoreans—thinkers who drew their inspiration from the philosopher and mathematician Pythagoras. It runs as follows:

I swear by Apollo Physician and Asclepius and Hygieia and Panaceia and all the gods and goddesses, making them my witnesses, that I will fulfil according to my ability and judgement this oath and covenant.

To hold him who has taught me this art as equal to my parents and to live my life in partnership with him, and if he is in need of money to give him a share of mine, and to regard his offspring as equal to my brothers in male lineage and to teach them this art—if they desire to learn it—without fee and covenant; to give a share of precepts and oral instruction and all the other learning to my sons and to the sons of him who has instructed me and to pupils who have signed the covenant and have taken an oath according to the medical law, but to no one else.

I will apply dietetic measures for the benefit of the sick according to my ability and judgement; I will keep them from harm and injustice.

I will neither give a deadly drug to anybody if asked for it, nor will I make a suggestion to this effect. Similarly I will not give to a woman an abortive remedy. In purity and holiness I will guard my life and my art.

I will not use the knife, not even on sufferers from stone, but will withdraw in favour of such men as are engaged in this work.

Whatever houses I may visit, I will come for the benefit of the sick, remaining free of all intentional injustice, of all mischief and in particular of sexual relations with both female and male persons, be they free or slaves.

What I may see or hear in the course of the treatment or even outside of the treatment in regard to the life of men, which on no account one must spread abroad, I will keep to myself holding such things shameful to be spoken about.

If I fulfil this oath and do not violate it, may it be granted to me to enjoy life and art, being honoured with fame among all men for all time to come; if I transgress it and swear falsely, may the opposite of all this be my lot. (From Ludwig Edelstein, *Ancient Medicine*, edited by

Oswei Temkin and C. Lillian Temkin (Baltimore: Johns Hopkins University Press, 1967).

Doctors frequently cite the oath, though very few medical schools now require their students to take it—and then only in an abbreviated and modified form.

human being A subject of experiences and of actions embodied in an organism of the species *Homo sapiens*. The existence of a human being is coextensive with the life of the corresponding subject. Thus, with brain death the life, and hence the existence, of the human being ceases, though if bodily life is sustained we may still be said to have a living human organism.

hypothermia A condition, caused by exposure to cold, in which the body is unable to maintain *core* (that is, internal) temperature at its proper level. Particularly common in poor elderly people living in their own homes, who may attempt to economize on heating.

hysteria A psychoneurosis associated with emotional excitability and various ostensibly physical symptoms that are ascribable to mental causes. (*Hustera*, in Greek, means womb: the ancient Greeks attributed hysterical symptoms, which seemed to them more common in women than in men, to the influence of the womb.)

implantation The process whereby the embryo attaches itself to the wall of the uterus; this usually happens at about fourteen days after conception.

informed consent Valid agreement to receive a particular type of treatment, given by the patient when he has received all the (available) information that is necessary to make a rational decision. Also applicable to a patient taking part in a clinical trial. In most American jurisdictions, courts have come to take the view that doctors should provide the patient with that level of information that a *reasonable patient* would consider adequate. English courts, in contrast, have not so far accepted this doctrine, preferring the standard of the *reasonable doctor* to that of the reasonable patient.

intuitionism A theory according to which moral principles, or at least the most fundamental ones, can, by someone possessed of the requisite moral insight, be seen to be true, without the need for argument, by exercising a faculty of moral intuition. On this view, we can simply see, for example, that lying is prima facie wrong, just as we can see that one plus one must equal two.

intuitive level According to the philosopher Richard Hare, there are two levels of moral thinking. In one, which he calls the *critical* level, one argues, along (preference) utilitarian lines, from first principles. In the other, which he calls the *intuitive* level, we act on the basis of rules, habits, dispositions of thought and character and the like, which may not be ostensibly utilitarian (or even consequentialist); according to Hare, however, these rules, dispositions, and so on (where valid) derive their ultimate justification from the fact that critical thinking shows that thinking in these terms has, for most practical purposes, a high utility. To try to decide every practical question by reasoning from first principles would be hopelessly time-consuming and would lend itself to all kinds of unconscious self-deception (making the utilitarian sums come out in one's own favour).

***in vitro* fertilization** Literally, fertilization in glass: the process whereby fertilization is achieved, outside the womb, by mixing sperm and one or more ova together in a glass dish. Hence 'test-tube babies', though one never in fact uses a test-tube for this purpose, but rather a flat dish known as a 'Petri dish'.

IUD Interuterine device: a contraceptive device, such as the coil, which stays in the uterus all the time. Such devices are generally thought, strictly speaking, to prevent not so much conception as the **implantation** of the fertilized ovum in the wall of the uterus.

justiciable A matter is justiciable if it is susceptible of being decided by a court of law.

leukaemia Literally, 'white blood'. A group of malignant blood disorders in which certain components of the blood undergo malignant change and proliferate.

normative Said of words that do not merely describe something but carry moral implications, particularly regarding appropriate conduct. 'Unjust' is an example of a normative term: to say that an action is unjust is not merely to describe it but to imply that it ought not, other things being equal, to be performed.

oncologist Specialist in tumours (including cancer).

palliative Said of a form of treatment that is designed to ameliorate the symptoms of a disease, but not to help cure it.

Parkinson's disease Progressive, degenerative condition involving loss of muscular control and a characteristic muscular tremor. Caused by the destruction of cells, in the *substantia nigra* of the brain, that produce the nerve-impulse transmitter substance, dopamine. May be partially controlled by a drug, L-dopa, that helps to compensate for the lack of naturally produced dopamine.

paternalism Literally, behaving towards someone as a father would towards his children; behaving towards someone in a way that does not respect his or her autonomy, for that person's own (supposed) good.

Paternalism characteristically involves making people's decisions for them or keeping certain information from them on the grounds that it would be better for them not to know.

person Sometimes used simply as a synonym for **human being**, but increasingly also (especially among philosophers) to mean a sentient being that has a concept of itself, and is capable of reflective, rational thought. On this usage a new-born baby would probably not count as a person, whereas an adult chimpanzee or dolphin might so count, as would intelligent beings on other planets, if any such exist.

prima facie To say that something is prima facie X is to say that it is to be taken as X in the absence of specific indications to the contrary. A prima facie duty, for example, is one that obliges one to act in a certain way, in the absence of a countervailing and more compelling duty to act otherwise.

primum non nocere Above all do no harm. A Latin tag derived from the **Hippocratic oath**.

Prisoners' Dilemma Two prisoners, assumed to be rational and purely self-interested, have been jointly involved in a bank robbery. The district attorney approaches each, offering a choice of confessing or not confessing. Each is told that, if neither confesses to the robbery, both prisoners will be convicted on the lesser charge of tax evasion, and will be sentenced to two years in gaol. If both confess, on the other hand, they will both be convicted of the bank robbery, and will each get six years in gaol. But if, finally, one confesses while the other does not, the one that confesses (having turned state's evidence) will get only one year in gaol, while the other gets ten. Each prisoner rationally ought to confess, since if the other confesses, it means getting six years rather than ten; and if the other does not confess, it means getting one year rather than two. Yet, paradoxically, the prisoners come off collectively worse by both doing this—getting six years each, whereas, if they had remained silent, they would only have got two. This is an example of what, in the *theory of games*, is known as a *non-zero sum game* (that is, one in which it is not true that what one participant gains the other automatically loses) with a *dominant strategy*, that is, a course of action that is best for each participant to choose, regardless of what the other participant does.

Some people have argued that the arms race has a similar logic. Each of the two superpowers can argue that, whether or not the other superpower steps up its armaments, it is best that it do so itself. For if the other side steps up its armaments, not to do so too would mean settling for military inferiority, which is perceived as being worse than approximate parity (albeit at a higher level of expenditure). If, on the other hand, the other side does not step up its armaments, to step up armaments would mean military superiority, which is perceived as being better than approximate parity (albeit at a lower level of expenditure). But if both sides step up their armaments, they will achieve approximate parity at a higher level of expenditure, whereas if neither side had stepped up its armaments, they would have had approximate parity at a lower level of expenditure, which both would agree to be preferable. This is obviously, at best, a gross oversimplification of the actual situation. In particular, as Bernard Williams points out, it ignores the time dimension: in a Prisoners' Dilemma-type game which repeatedly recurs, it is rational and possible for each side to adopt the *co-operative* strategy (not confessing or not stepping up armaments) in the hope that the other participant will follow suit; a principle of tit-for-tat (copying what the other participant did last time round) may be used to encourage the other participant to adopt the co-operative strategy.

prognosis   The likely or predicted outcome or future course of a disease.

prophylactic   Said of a drug or other form of treatment that is designed to prevent some condition developing.

radiotherapy   Treatment of malignant disease with X-rays or by the implantation of radioactive metals, such as cobalt.

real essence   A term due to the philosopher John Locke (1632–1704) and given new currency in consequence of the work of the contemporary American philosopher Saul Kripke. The real essence of something is what makes it the thing that it is, a set of attributes that it must, of necessity, possess if it is to exist at all. Thus, the real essence of gold is its being composed of atoms with atomic number 79. Anything with a different atomic constitution, however like gold it was, could not actually be gold. Likewise, it has been argued that having the particular biological parents that he does is part of the real essence of a human being: that very same human being could not have existed and yet had different parents.

rule utilitarianism   A form of utilitarianism according to which an action is to be judged right or wrong, not according to its consequences in the particular case, but rather according to whether it is or is not enjoined by those rules, adoption of which would be expected to have the best consequences. Thus, if keeping one's promises is judged to be a good rule, in the sense that the consequences of people adopting it are judged good, in utilitarian terms, then it may sometimes, for a rule utilitarian, be best to keep a promise, even where the consequences of so doing would seem less good than the consequences of breaking it. There is growing agreement among philosophers that this is a confused doctrine;

Hare's theory of intuitive and critical levels of thinking might be seen as a clearer and more defensible statement of the insight that underlies it.

schizophrenia A psychotic condition characterized by loss of contact with reality and the disintegration of the personality. Symptoms range from hallucinations and delusions to a state of stupor, as in *catatonic schizophrenia*. Frequently confused, in ordinary speech, with the much rarer (and possibly non-existent) condition of *multiple personality*.

self-awareness or **self-consciousness** A being is self-aware if it is (a) *conscious* or **sentient** and (b) has a concept of itself; that is, is able to reflect upon its own actions, states of awareness, and so forth.

sentience Something is sentient if it has the capacity for *consciousness*; that is, if it has experiences. Sentience and consciousness must not be confused either with the capacity to respond to stimuli, which does not logically entail sentience, or with **self-awareness** or *reflective consciousness*, which imply, respectively, the possession of a concept of self and the capacity for reflective thought.

sine qua non Literally, 'without which not'. A *sine qua non*, for example of a crime, is something that is essential to the commission of the crime, or alternatively an essential part of the cause—some event or state of affairs without which it would not have occurred.

surrogate motherhood or **surrogacy** The practice whereby a woman bears a child to term with the aim of handing it over to another woman. The term is used to describe both (a) cases in which pregnancy is induced by artificial (or natural) insemination, usually by the husband or male partner of the woman who is to receive the child, and (b) the practice, sometimes also known as *womb leasing* in which an embryo is produced by *in vitro* **fertilization**, usually with an ovum taken from the woman who wants the child, and then transferrd to the womb of another woman who will hand it over to the genetic mother when it is born.

therapeutic research Clinical research that is incidental to the primary aim of helping the patient, and from which the patient is likely to benefit. *Non-therapeutic research*, by contrast, is research that has as its primary purpose the acquisition of knowledge.

transitive relation A relation is said to be transitive if, given that it holds between A and B and also between B and C, it follows that it must also hold between A and C. An example of a transitive relation would be *taller than*: if Tom is taller than Dick and Dick is taller than Harriet, it follows that Tom is taller than Harriet.

undifferentiated See **differentiation**.

utilitarianism A form of **consequentialism** according to which the goodness or badness of happenings or states of affairs is to be gauged entirely on the basis of the aggregate benefit that is conferred on the affected parties. *Classical utilitarianism* equates benefit with happiness, usually thought of as the positive balance of enjoyment over suffering; *preference utilitarianism* equates benefit with desire fulfilment.

INDEX

OXFORD

MORE OXFORD PAPERBACKS

Details of a selection of other books follow. A complete list of Oxford Paperbacks, including The World's Classics, Twentieth-Century Classics, OPUS, Past Masters, Oxford Authors, Oxford Shakespeare, and Oxford Paperback Reference, is available in the UK from the General Publicity Department, Oxford University Press, Walton Street, Oxford, OX2 6DP.

In the USA, complete lists are available from the Paperbacks Marketing Manager, Oxford University Press, 200 Madison Avenue, New York, NY 10016.

BETRAYERS OF THE TRUTH

Fraud and Deceit in Science

William Broad and Nicholas Wade

Why are scientists tempted to cheat? What leads a man who has devoted his life to the pursuit of the truth to fabricate evidence? Do rhetoric and propaganda play as large a role in science as they do in politics, law, and religion? *Betrayers of the Truth* analyses how the lure of fame and big money can lead scientists to abandon the ideals of their profession. Drawing on examples from astronomy, physics, biology, and medicine, the authors discuss scientific fraud as a historical phenomenon, perpetrated by men as separated in time as Ptolemy and Mendel, Newton and Sir Cyril Burt. They also explore fraud as a modern problem, endemic in the huge research factories which are part and parcel of modern scientific investigation.

'a highly responsible and well-argued contribution to the sociology of science'. Peter Medawar, *London Review of Books*

SHOULD THE BABY LIVE?

The Problem of Handicapped Infants

Helga Kuhse and Peter Singer

This book concerns itself with both the practical and philosophical issues of allowing certain handicapped babies to die. The authors' conclusions are not absolutist in any direction: rather they believe that careful rational examination of the admittedly complex issues—which they present clearly and by way of actual examples—an lead to responsible decisions of different kinds in different cases.

Studies in Bioethics

THE REPRODUCTION REVOLUTION

New Ways of Making Babies

Peter Singer & Deane Wells

On 25 July 1978 in Oldham, Lancashire, Louise Brown was born. She was the first test-tube baby, and with her began a new era in childbirth. Now, five years after this event, *in vitro* fertilization and other technological advances are brining hope to infertile couples in clinics throughout the world.

The authors of this accessible new book argue that it is high time we faced up to the complex ethical problems of the reproduction revolution. They explore the new processes through the eyes of both the doctor, and of the potential parents. They also look to the future when ectogenesis (development outside the womb), cloning, sex selection, and genetic engineering may become commonplace.

Studies in Bioethics